Printed in the United States of America
ISBN: 979-8-218-29302-4

The cover image is my original drawing called "The Journey." The sailing canoe represents the journey through life and into the great beyond. As the canoe moves out to sea, it fades gently into the stars.

My Hawaiian ancestors were skillful navigators who traveled the oceans, and I have adapted that heritage to my calling to help patients and their families gracefully navigate their own journeys through the end-of-life process in hospice.

DEMYSTIFYING HOSPICE
The Secrets to Navigating
End-of-Life Care

Barbara Petersen, RN

*This book is dedicated to the patients and their families
who welcomed me into their lives and allowed me the privilege
of caring for them at such a sacred time.*

Table of Contents

Introduction

Why Read This Book?

I have chosen to write a different kind of hospice book—one that helps you know all about hospice before you need it.

These pages contain specific details, precise information about the business, the physical decline a patient might experience, and the medication management given to relieve symptoms prior to death.

A book like this helps the family and caregivers of hospice patients know what to expect during the process. It allows caregivers to better help the patients as they grieve their loss of function. It also helps caregivers become more aware of how to anticipate their own grief. In addition, this book will help all professionals involved in the provision of hospice services learn more about what it entails and do their jobs better. It may even help some people in these professions decide whether they want to get, or stay with, a job in hospice.

Other books exist to offer lofty, feel-good, emotionally driven tales about hospice and stories about the amazing scope of the hospice process experienced by patients, families, and staff. Differently, this book describes the "nuts and bolts" of giving care to hospice patients. This is the story I am reporting after

20 years as a hospice nurse, so I address some uncomfortable truths about it and the business side of it.

What You Will Encounter

Note that each chapter is a stand-alone topic and can be read in any order, so you can choose what is most applicable to you and your situation.

Chapter 1 briefly recounts the history of how the hospice program was started and became supported by insurance and Medicare. I tell my perception about the struggles and the creativity of the nurses, doctors, and many agencies involved that it took to develop this amazing program.

Chapter 2 outlines who the players are and who does what, from the legal aspects to the clinical staff of a hospice agency.

Chapter 3 delivers several clinical scenarios that help the reader learn about the major shifts in patients' capabilities that trigger massive changes in their disease trajectory.

Chapter 4 relates how medications are used and explains the legal and practical aspects of the uses of medications.

Chapter 5 details the symptoms and interventions during the dying process itself.

Chapter 6 takes the reader through the hospice process from beginning to end, from the decision to use hospice to the sacred time after the death.

Chapter 7 offers a tribute to the nurses, recognizing their extraordinary passion and abilities nurtured in their schools, universities, and jobs that prepare them for this very special, holistic kind of nursing care.

What Exactly Is Hospice Care?

Hospice care is a program that offers help from experts in the medical field who understand how to manage the symptoms of illness and facilitate the dying process. These professionals do everything possible to reduce uncomfortable symptoms while the patient's body is declining. This is done in an aggressive manner because time is of the essence for anyone in distress.

Hospice care is available before, during, and after a person transitions to death. It is available to those who have a life-limiting illness, have stopped curative treatments, and have been given a six-month prognosis.

Hospice care differs from palliative care in which a patient may or may not have a life-limiting illness and the scope of services is to manage symptoms that, in many cases, lead to a cure. This service also is limited to the attention of a medical doctor and/or a nurse practitioner.

In contrast, hospice programs involve professionals from multiple disciplines who visit the patient and the family. The focus is on quality of life and comfort rather than curing the illness. With the goal of providing the best quality of life and comfort, any tests or treatments involving the painful use of a needle are avoided. Any symptoms that can be managed immediately without tests are treated.

Managing a person through illness and death focuses on creating a peaceful passing that is symptom-free, in great part due to the careful administration of medications. Many think that hospice includes a nurse who is at the house doing the care for as many hours or days as the family requests, but that is not the case. Nurses visit a few days a week.

Dispelling Myths

Unfortunately, not all experiences with hospice are seen as positive, and critical stories unfortunately have been believed without checking them out. Following are the most common myths, which are other significant reasons for writing this book:

+ Morphine kills.
+ Palliative care is better.
+ A nurse is in-home 24/7 free of charge.
+ All medications are stopped.
+ People choke to death.

To help dispel misinformation, I offer brief explanations about the errors in these dangerously perpetuated myths.

Morphine Kills

The most common example of a hospice myth is about the use of morphine. Some report that morphine caused their loved one's death because they noted that the person died soon after receiving a dose.

There is a well-known phenomenon about comfort and dying: Dying is a very difficult process unless the patient is comfortable. The reality is that morphine provides symptom relief, and, when the person is comfortable, they can let go. A person's spirit does not have an easy time transitioning when the patient is in pain or agitated or having trouble breathing or dealing with psychological stress.

Dispelling myths like this can help the world understand that medications always are given carefully. It is against the law to overmedicate a patient to facilitate a death. All hospice staff take this responsibility very seriously.

If you have questions about the use of morphine and death resulting soon after, please read on and consider the variability and scope of this issue and what the person you are thinking about may have experienced.

From my 20 years as a hospice nurse, I can tell you all the ways that this phenomenon was interpreted, understood, explained, justified, and rationalized by family and/or the hospice staff. Following is a list of many of the possible things that might have happened between the time the medication was given and the time the patient died. You might think of others.

"They gave the medication...
AND THEN...
the patient died!"

But what happened during the IN BETWEEN time?

- The patient's pain was relieved.

- The patient's breathing was no longer labored.

- The patient's anxiety was reduced.

- The patient's agitation went away.

- The patient saw a deceased relative welcome them.

- The patient realized they didn't have to be afraid.

- The patient was welcomed by a figure central to their religion and was not afraid.

- The patient recognized that they were forgiven for all their transgressions.

- The patient's spirit let go of the need to stay alive for someone else.

- The patient took the hand of their deceased spouse, child, parent, or lover and left with them.

- The patient reviewed their life's happy moments.

- The patient reviewed their life's sad moments but saw them as lessons learned.

- The patient realized they didn't have to be afraid of the medicine.

- The patient saw the bright white light that so many others have reported and felt at peace.

- The patient recognized that all their family members would be fine and that their dying was not going to be a crisis for them.

- The patient recognized that their family members have been fantastic about ensuring the quality of their life during the dying process, and when they are gone, the family will not have to do that any longer.

- The patient accepted their desire and ability to let go.

- **THEN they died!**

I hope this list will help families and patients reduce their fears about morphine. I also hope that if, and when, they are asked about it, they will feel comfortable sharing some of these ideas. This is further addressed in Chapters 4 and 5.

Palliative Care Is Better

Palliative care should not be chosen just because patients or their families are uncomfortable with the idea of hospice care. Palliative care is its own specialty.

Dying patients do not start with palliative care and then decide later that they are more accepting and will begin hospice care. If a patient needs aggressive symptom management that a palliative care professional can provide and their diagnosis is not terminal, they begin palliative care.

When a person has a terminal diagnosis, they should not waste any time with the limited care available from palliative care. They should start hospice care right away so they can get all the services available to them. This is covered in detail in Chapters 1 and 2.

A Nurse Is In-Home 24/7 Free of Charge

As much as health agencies would love to have nurses help your family through the entire time that hospice care is needed, there simply are not enough nurses in the world to cover that need. If you have heard of that happening, it was either a situation in which a family was able to afford a private duty nurse or the patient was in critical condition and, for a short period of time, nurses did come to do 24/7 care. However, the correct name for that is continuous care.

As much as we empathize with the family's needs and love for the patient, agencies do not have the money to choose to cover the care for one patient and not another. There are not enough nurses nor enough money to do it any other way. It breaks our hearts every time we have to correct this misunderstanding because we know the time and effort, love and devotion, privilege and honor, and physical and emotional toll that hospice care can take on everyone.

When a family thinks they will be given all that professional help free of charge and then they find out it is not available, it often becomes a crisis. If you ever hear someone talking about hospice that way, correct them immediately and save everyone the shock and dismay they will feel later. This is further explained in Chapter 2.

All Medications Are Stopped

In recent years, due to rising costs, some agencies now cover fewer medications. The agencies are required to cover the medications that manage the dying symptoms, but they are not required to cover any over-the-counter supplements or medications taken for diagnoses unrelated to the terminal diagnosis. This subject is covered in detail in Chapter 4.

People Choke to Death

A particular symptom happens to many patients who are actively dying. When they are no longer aware of the need to swallow or clear their throat, the patient's own saliva and the very small amount of oral liquid medications can collect in the back of the throat and cause a gurgling sound. In the old days, that was termed a "death rattle." Most of the time, medications can dry that fluid and stop the symptom, but, regardless, this fluid does not cause them to choke to death. This subject is covered in detail in Chapter 5.

While the goal of this book is to explain what hospice is and what hospice is not, it is also to tell the story of what happens while a person is dying. Explaining the patterns will help the patient and their family as well as the nursing home staff know what to do. This information is helpful to anyone wanting to be prepared ahead of time for the experience.

Chapter 1:
A Brief History of
Hospice Services

Hospice care started in England in 1948 when Dame Cycily Saunders fell in love with a man who was dying. She was a nurse, social worker, doctor, and writer. She began to focus on comfort and quality-of-life care and urging families to take people out of the hospital and let them die more comfortably at home.

Following are some significant dates and events that show how long ago this wonderful program was initiated. It has taken quite a while to come to the complexity of services that are available today.

1967: St. Christopher's Hospice was opened in the United Kingdom.

1969: Elisabeth Kübler-Ross wrote *On Death and Dying*. Through sample interviews and conversations, she gives readers a better understanding of how imminent death affects the patient, the professionals who serve that patient, and the patient's family with the aim of bringing hope to all who are involved.

1978: The National Hospice and Palliative Care Organization (NHPCO) was established to promote hospice and palliative care.

1983: The Medicare hospice benefit was established under the Reagan Administration.

1993: Hospice was included as a nationally guaranteed benefit under President Clinton's healthcare reform proposal.

Hospice care is now an accepted part of the U.S. healthcare continuum. It became as well-known and effective as it is today because of very courageous and intelligent nursing directors, doctors, and administrators. They trained their nurses about anatomy, physiology, and pharmacology so well that these nurses became groundbreakers as the teachers of many local doctors.

Many doctors resisted the change to embracing hospice care because they had been educated and trained to cure the disease while this new specialty was focused instead on comfort until death.

In the 10 years after the nationally guaranteed benefit was established—a few years after we turned the corner into this new century—doctors began to accept that patients who declared their intention to die at home deserved to have the support to obtain the quality of life they wanted instead of meeting resistance while facing their lifechanging illness.

As patients began to get that respect, and the doctors learned about the successes of in-home hospice, the century during which most people felt it necessary to be in a hospital to die came to a close. Medical professionals were encouraging people to remain at home instead so they might feel safe and comfortable dying in their own bed, which actually had been the standard just a century before.

Agency Backing

To better advertise hospice care, nurses and marketing staff from these newly formed agencies hung around hospitals, nursing homes, and doctor's offices to spread the word about all the benefits of hospice programs. They reported on the systems for treating patients in their own homes, in nursing homes, and even in hospitals.

Agencies representing the different diagnoses (such as the American Heart Association and American Cancer Society) spoke up for people's rights to object to further curative care and started supporting both the person's opportunity and right to choose to remain at home to die.

Then even more medical areas and the funeral professions began to pay attention, and soon professional medical organizations, emergency services, coroners, funeral homes, and crematoriums all gave authority to the hospice staff to declare a death in a home setting instead of calling 911 to summon first responders.

Legal Support

Gaining the trust of all legal parties to protect patients from unnecessary trauma by cardiopulmonary resuscitation (CPR) came with a caveat. They wanted to reduce the risks that, when hospice staff declared a patient dying at home, there would be no suspicion of anything illegal or illicit going on. So, they initiated a new rule and a process called DO NOT CALL 911, and they instituted a requirement that hospice patients should have a DNR. A DNR (Do Not Resuscitate) is a form signed by the patient or patient's legal Power of Attorney for Health Care (POAHC) and a doctor, stipulating that no CPR should be performed if the patient becomes unresponsive and unable to present a pulse or respiration.

If a patient's caregiver does not have a DNR form to hand to an emergency medical service worker, the medic or EMT (emergency medical technician) will perform CPR when called to a home where someone has no pulse. CPR is the process of trying to resuscitate the heart and breathing by forcefully pressing on the chest and pushing air into the lungs through the mouth.

When a death is expected and accepted, doing CPR on anyone, especially a frail elderly person, is rather brutal because it can potentially break their ribs. As such, everyone must have the required legal paperwork to protect the patient, the family, and the emergency medical services. The use of DNR forms and the admonition of "NO 911" were critical to developing hospice programs. This has all taken time, but the systems work very well today.

Care Collaboration to Effect Change

Developing this special care also offered the opportunity for all the primary occupations—registered nurse (RN), social worker (SW), chaplain or spiritual counselor (SC), certified nursing assistant (CNA), nurse practitioner (NP), medical doctor (MD), volunteers, administrators, marketers, and other skilled nursing facility staff—to be even more creative and explore how to set the environment in facilities to be as homelike as possible for both the patients and their families. They collaborated by making suggestions to families and facilities regarding the furniture and decorations, providing extra beds for family, allowing 24/7 visiting hours, offering chapels and food for visitors, and establishing routines that all help manage a "peaceful death" with compassionate care for the family as well.

Medication Administration

Learning how to aggressively resolve the symptoms of dying was, of course, a new concept for all the medical professions. Hospitals have pharmacies that can deliver a variety of medications in various forms within hours. So, for the home patients, specialized neighborhood pharmacies were created to serve them within hours. This resulted in much less suffering for patients, fewer calls to doctor's offices, and calmer families.

Some pharmacies have become specialists in hospice care, and, along with doctors, have created new combinations and forms of drugs for ease of administration. These compounding pharmacies created medications as patches, gels, and liquids instead of injections so caregivers would be able to administer medications less painfully under the consideration that relief of symptoms is the primary goal. Pharmacies also hired drivers to deliver medications to patients the same day, and doctors wrote orders with more flexibility about the doses and their timing. This allowed more aggressive treatment that was properly supported by research but new in the home setting.

Hospice Homes

The collaborative teams also created freestanding hospice "homes" called In-Patient Units. Some were located in wings of a hospital or in nursing homes. The rooms here are more like normal bedrooms without all the hospital paraphernalia, noise, and other patients.

Now, fewer people stay in hospitals to die. Although more patients are able to be in their homes, the majority of hospice patients are in nursing homes. This is truer in the United States than in other countries, where the culture of the nuclear family still includes multiple generations who remain at home until they die.

Financial Business Implications

Because of Centers for Medicare & Medicaid Services (CMS) rules, accepting the reality that people die clearly has been more difficult for nursing home administrators. It has become unfortunate but true that financial considerations often determine why and when a patient gets into hospice. For some reason, nursing homes still consider it a blight on their record if someone dies while living there!

To reduce the percentage of that unfortunate evaluation statistic, when a patient begins to decline, nursing homes will hurry up and get them admitted to hospice. As such, the last bills for that patient, and the facility's statistics for the month, show that Medicare, or another private insurance, paid the bill from that hospice budget line item. This shows that the patient's death was anticipated and not potentially seen as the fault of the nursing home staff. This is a holdover from the "curative" model of care.

The truth is that in-house deaths affect future payments by CMS. Many times, the patient's death occurs within 24 hours, but the nursing home considers it a winning decision. The hospice agency often delivers five days' worth of care in 24 hours that is not truly covered by the amount of money they are paid by CMS. But the hospice caregivers and the nursing home know a good service was provided, so that reality keeps everyone going.

Finding the Right Home Health and Hospice Agency

Today, all the many home health and hospice agencies, as with anything, are competing for your business. When you search for an agency, look carefully and read about their programs to know exactly which services are available and who pays for them.

Palliative Care

Palliative care is a very valuable service, but it is its own specialty. Someone can have that support with or without home health or hospice agency care. A hospice website may explain palliative care, making it look like all the services listed are included in both palliative and hospice care, but they are not.

Palliative care programs include visits by an advanced practice registered nurse or medical doctor to help manage symptoms that may or may not be life-threatening. A person does not need to be in hospice to get palliative care. The aggressive symptom management available from a nurse practitioner in a palliative care program is for people in their homes, nursing homes, or hospitals who have complicated and hard-to-manage side effects from a disease process. The patient's disease does not have to be life-threatening; they just need a nurse practitioner who works with a medical doctor to come and visit and get orders for medications or treatments that other doctors may not have thought about.

Check your benefits for the coverage of this CMS- and private insurance–supported program. Also check your pharmacy coverage to know about the cost of the medications. All the other specialties available in hospice care are not provided for palliative care. No one else will be coming to give care and support. It's important to know the difference.

Vigil Care

Vigil care may or may not be offered by an agency. Many families think that someone needs to be with their loved one at the time of death, so agencies may offer this. Look carefully to see whether the agency specifies who covers that cost and if it is actually available.

Paying for Care

Agencies may provide home health as well as hospice care, and Medicare pays 80% for home health and 100% for most of the things needed for hospice. Due to rising costs, some agencies now may cover fewer medications, but not the symptom-management ones required for the terminal diagnosis. Some agencies have a copay for five-day respite care.

Today, the agencies must ensure that each patient meets strict criteria to be admitted for hospice care. Just 10 years ago, many people were literally dying of old age in convalescent care with a diagnosis of "debility unspecified" without any critical illness yet still spending five years obtaining hospice services.

In 2014, Medicare got wise to this and decided to remove that category from the list of diagnoses it would cover. Then it got even stricter in all the disease categories about how much more debilitated one had to be to qualify. Medicare realized that the taxpayer was paying for many more months and years of care than anticipated and that the system needed revision. It didn't seem so at the time because families did not have the funds to pay for all the supplies and equipment, but it was a good thing.

Home health criteria also were examined and modified. That issue increased the likelihood of a patient being transferred to a nursing home.

The bottom line is that there are limitations in business, as any business owner knows. There is no limit to the number of days a person can receive services, but they must continue clinically to need the kind of care it provides.

Benefits of In-Home Care

Hospice care can be done in the person's home, and this is the ideal situation for the nurse to be confident about the family's education, training, and follow through. When only the immediate family and hired caregivers need to be educated about the schedules for staff visits, a patient's diagnoses and symptoms, the medication list, how to give all the medications and do the treatments, and know how to work the equipment and supplies, organization is easier. But not all families can afford to hire the necessary staff or have enough family members to provide the 24/7 attendance required at the end of a person's life. As such, nursing home placement is arranged with Medicaid for those who qualify.

The Choice

All hospitals and nursing homes have their favorite agencies. In some cases, the hospice agency and nursing home are part of the same corporation. However, you can choose any agency you want. Most agencies cover several different counties, are independent, and all go to the same facilities.

Now, hospice care is well-known to most staff (clinical as well as administrative), so an experienced facility nurse will know to expect the delivery of special medications and equipment, the discontinuation of certain orders, and that a CNA will come twice a week to bathe the patient, which can be a relief for their own daily scheduling. Thanks to the education from hospice staff, they know to call the agency for the changes they have come to recognize.

For several years, the hospice specialty has been an elective in both nursing schools and residencies for medical students. Having them trained has helped raise awareness of what a decline in a patient's condition toward being a hospice patient looks like, and patients, families, and facilities are benefitting from hospice services earlier.

Although hospice has been a known entity in the United States since *On Death and Dying* was published here in America in 1969, what we've learned is that until someone encounters the experience in their life, many things about it remain a mystery.

Chapter 2:
How the System Works

In the introduction, two topics that have become myths were briefly presented. Here they will be thoroughly addressed.

1. **A nurse comes to the home and does all the care for us, right?**

Wrong! The only kind of hospice nursing care in which you will have a nurse stay in the home 24/7, paid by the insurance or CMS, to provide the care to the patient is a service and level of care within hospice programs called continuous care. It is for patients whose symptoms are out of control, and it is very rare and short term.

Routine hospice care is the category for 99.99% of patients, and it does not include having a nurse in the home for the duration of the person's life.

2. **Palliative care is like hospice care, so I will choose to do that because I'm uncomfortable with the idea of "hospice."**

Wrong! If the complexity of hospice care is what is needed, palliative care will not suffice. Palliative care is a pathway of care typically comprising a nurse practitioner working in collaboration with a physician. These nurses with masters degrees are specially trained professionals who make visits to palliative care patients to prescribe medication and treatments or follow up to manage the treatment of symptoms for as long as the patient needs them. The term "curative intent" is highly applicable in the realm of palliative care, but it is not the focus of hospice care. In palliative care, patients may or may not have a life-limiting illness, and patients can continue to seek curative treatments, such as chemotherapy, radiation therapy, blood transfusions, and IV treatments.

In some instances, palliative care is used as a steppingstone to hospice care only because the patient's treatments did not cure the illness and so hospice care is then needed. But as previously noted, not all patients receiving palliative care are suffering from a life-limiting illness.

This program was not designed as a steppingstone for those who fear the term and concept of "hospice," so a family should not choose palliative care simply because they are emotionally uncomfortable and know the patient is dying. If a family member is uncomfortable about the term hospice or the reality of dying, they need a lot of education and emotional support. It is unfortunate that some families demand that the hospice staff avoid using the term "hospice" in the home of a patient. They even ask that nametags with the agency identified be removed or taped over.

The misconceptions people have regarding palliative and hospice care often are about the services offered. In hospice, multiple disciplines provide services to the patient and family, and those are described in the rest of this chapter.

Organizations and Staff Responsibilities

CMS

CMS stands for the Centers for Medicare & Medicaid Services. Medicare and Medicaid, as well as most private insurance companies, pay a daily fee to hospice agencies. The amount of money depends on the level of care that is provided: Routine, Continuous, General In-Patient, and Respite.

At one time, no copay or bill was sent to patients and their families under Medicare and Medicaid, but in the last few years, expenses have risen so high that agencies now have an option to cover everything or only selected medications. An Advanced Beneficiary Notice (ABN) is given to the family that lists what the agency does not cover. Medicare Part D may bill the agency if there is any disagreement about what should be covered. The required symptom-management medications may include a $5 copayment, but many agencies do not charge for these medications. The Medicare Part D funds may cover some additional medications, but the patient and family most likely will cover the cost of any over-the-counter supplements if they choose to continue using them. Medicare does not cover room and board if you get hospice care in your home or if the patient lives in a nursing home. You also may have a copay for a portion of respite care.

Definitely check the policies if you have private insurance. A decade ago, private insurance lagged way behind CMS in covering hospice services. They now have caught up a lot, but they may require more of a copay.

Routine Care is the first level of care. Let's say, hypothetically, that CMS pays $200 per day for routine hospice care. That money needs to cover all the administration and staff salaries, the business overhead, equipment, supplies, and medication needed by the patient. In the first five days, visits will be made to the patient and/or the family by four of the six clinicians.

The agency pays fees to the equipment and supply companies and the pharmacy and pays for medications the patient takes. The agencies cover many things, but agencies simply cannot afford to provide some pieces of specialized equipment. They will provide a safe and effective product, but it just may not be what the patient or family preferred.

For example, if the patient needs the Imogen air concentrator, the agencies may provide a portable tank on wheels instead. The Imogen is a very lightweight, backpack-style portable oxygen concentrator used by mobile people who need oxygen all the time but usually do not need hospice care. It is provided in home health agency care, but usually not in hospice care.

The agencies must follow the regulations stipulated by CMS because their daily payment is all that most agencies have available to pay the bills. The portable oxygen tank for the patient to use while outside the home is about three feet tall and secured in a carrier on wheels. An oxygen concentrator is a machine on wheels that is the patient's primary source of additional oxygen. The tank functions well, is portable, fits into a car, and can be placed in a closet to be out of the way at home. It's the emergency backup tank if the electricity goes out and the concentrator cannot work. Some patients don't like it, but if they don't qualify for the Imogen, it cannot be provided. We must ensure that this oxygen source is available in case of a power outage, and the tanks are perfect for that.

Some agencies are very large and have a donor base that gives them more latitude to provide extra devices, but that is rare. It really is important that the agencies follow the CMS rules. They take fraud and abuse very seriously, which is why they perform audits. Some agencies have been taken to court and fined six-figure penalties for violating the rules.

Routine-level care will have the registered nurse (RN) and the certified nursing assistant (CNA) come as often as necessary to meet the needs of the patient. It's common to have two visits by both the RN and CNA each week. A social worker and chaplain may visit weekly, but more often, they visit monthly, depending on the requests of the patient and family. As the patient's condition changes, commonly referred to as decline, the frequency of visits by all staff will increase.

Continuous Care is the second level of nursing care. It is very uncommon and is a special service during which an RN stays 24 hours every day to provide all the care to the patient, whether that is in a private home, an assisted living facility, or skilled nursing facility (SNF). At times, a patient will be transferred to either a hospital for General In-Patient (GIP) care or a freestanding facility known as an In-Patient Unit (IPU). In those circumstances, the nurses in those facilities do the 24/7 nursing care.

CMS and private insurance pay much more per day for this ICU-type of clinical care for the patient. Understanding the conditions that qualify for continuous care is very important. This 24/7 in-home care is provided when the patient has uncontrolled symptoms of pain, shortness of breath, nausea and vomiting, or agitation.

Two nurses each work 12-hour shifts in the home for specific care of the patient and support for the family. They do not provide assistance to any other member of the family or clean any space outside the immediate area where the care for the patient is given. A family member or hired homemaker is expected to be in the home as well, and that person will care for any dependent children or other adults needing care.

The continuous care nurses do not perform any household management while they are on duty. They are present to do continuous assessments of the patient and report those to the family, the agency, and the doctors. With this service, nurses are in the home for as many days as it takes to bring the symptoms under control. When it is suddenly necessary to manage more than one symptom, this can take from a few days to several to determine the right combination and doses of medications. With only one symptom, it may only take a day. In that instance, the agency may allow another day or two to ensure that the medications are working and that the family is set up to manage the care. Then the continuous care is stopped, and the family resumes doing everything.

If the nurse assesses that the patient's death is imminent, the continuous care may continue. This only happens if the patient still needs skilled hourly assessments about which medications and dosages to give. If the patient's physical care and medication routine can be handled by the family, continuous care will be discontinued.

Having the family assume full care for their dying loved one is common. Many families decide to handle the care and not to have a stranger in the home at that time. Being able to do every aspect of care for their loved one during those last days and hours is considered a sacred privilege. Even if they were very afraid of doing so just days before, many people will become capable after excellent teaching by the nurse and support from other staff as they honor a patient's wishes.

It is simply not possible to provide a nurse in every home to manage the care of every hospice patient whether they are actively dying or not. Instead, it is our job to teach the family or staff how to manage their care and medications. Some families do that more easily than others, but for those families that find it too difficult, the solution is either to hire caregivers to come to the home or transfer the patient to an SNF.

There are many caregiver agencies the family can hire to obtain the needed level of care. The family interviews the prospective caregiver—sometimes with the help of a member of the hospice team—and the family hires the caregiver and pays their salary. Throughout the time a person is in hospice, the nurse, social worker, aide, and chaplain will be watching to note any dramatic changes in their condition that warrant continuous care. And, of course, they will watch for the expected decline that reveals that the family needs more caregivers. By knowing the family structure and assets, they will make suggestions and help assess their needs as well as train additional caregivers.

General In-Patient (GIP) is the next level of care. This is continuous care provided in a hospital. When a patient has unmanaged symptoms that require hourly assessments and administration of medications or treatments, the daily fee from CMS is higher. If a person already is in the hospital, there is a billing system change from routine care to hospice GIP care, and the nursing staff provides this higher level of care. A patient can be transferred to a hospital or a freestanding In-Patient Unit (IPU) from an SNF or home. Some hospice agencies own a freestanding facility/IPU, but most agencies do not, so they utilize the GIP status in a local hospital as needed.

The hospice agency gets this care started and writes the orders, then the hospital or IPU staff nurses and aides provide the care. The registered nurse/case manager for the agency visits daily to make sure the hospice agency attention is clear and orders are followed as well as to assess whether the patient is comfortable, get new orders as needed, and report back to the family. The same rules apply for how long continuous care is given in that setting or in the home. As soon as the symptoms are managed, the patient resumes routine care. That can be given with the patient staying in the hospital or being transferred to a facility or home where they lived before and where the family or facility staff resume doing the care.

Respite Care is the last level of care. This is available when the family needs to take a short break. This gives them a respite from doing the 24-hour care by having the patient transported to a nursing facility. Care is then done in an SNF for five days at a time and is available every few months. The fee to the agency, which pays the SNF, is higher than for routine care; in recent years some agencies have asked the family for a copay. The patient is transported by ambulance, which hospice pays for, and the care is provided by the SNF staff. The hospice agency staff continues their visits that week as if the patient were at home. If the family needs respite for more than five days, or they need it sooner than the rules permit, the family will have to absorb some, if not all, of the costs.

The Hospice Team

Every hospice team member will make you feel like you're the only person in the world to them. The sincerity of truly listening to each person comes from their compassionate understanding of how difficult and scary this time in your life feels. It is their intention to help you trust them as they offer their skills and provide options to you that can make this entire process less difficult. The team has lots of experience knowing what physical and emotional changes the patient will go through based on the diagnosis. When there are changes that they notice during their visits, they communicate with each other daily about additional medical or spiritual care needed by the patient or the family members. All staff make their own schedules because they care for several home and skilled nursing facility (SNF) patients in a day.

Time is of the essence in hospice care. Making additional visits (even in the middle of the night), obtaining medications the same day, or changing medications or dosages in the same day are common in hospice care versus what you will find in allopathic medical care. A nurse practitioner is more likely to make a visit to the patient than the medical doctor/medical director, but even that is rare. The skills and confidence of the nurse practitioner and registered nurse/case manager are such that their reports to the medical doctor and nursing supervisor are trusted.

Registered Nurses (RNs) are the case managers (CMs) who make or break a good experience in hospice care. Along with the medical director, the RNs determine which medications and treatments are needed to keep the patient comfortable. RNs educate all parties involved about the patient's care and how to administer medications and treatments. Visits are made once or twice a week, depending on the patient's needs, until there is a decline. The visits increase to seven days a week for a patient who is actively dying.

Certified Nursing Assistants (CNAs) come twice a week to give the patient a shower or bed bath, as determined by the patient's ability to move and stand or sit safely. An experienced CNA can assess a patient's status very well, and their reports to the RN/CM about skin, pain, and decline are critically important. They do a full skin assessment during the bath, and they may make recommendations about turning the patient in bed more frequently and then teach the family about that process. They can teach about their care to other caregivers and family members in the home to ensure that the care is being done properly and safely.

CNAs communicate with the patient in such a way that they know if psychological changes are occurring with the patient and the family members. They change linens weekly (or more often as needed) and clean the space around the patient's bed and nightstand as well as make sure the patient is changed, clean, and has water nearby. They may feed the patient if they are able to be at the SNF or patient's home during mealtime.

Often the compassion and kindness expressed by the CNA, who is so intimately involved with the patient, is the most impressive. Their name will be the one that the patient and family will remember the most as time goes by.

Medical Social Workers (MSWs) assess the readiness of the patient and family for what they are facing. Grieving is complicated and already will have started before admission to hospice. The MSW provides emotional support and practical assistance to the patient, family, and caregivers. They evaluate the financial and caregiving needs to determine whether a transfer to an SNF or hiring additional caregivers in the home might be needed. They know whether Veterans services are available, as appropriate. They understand the regulations of who pays what in SNF and know when applying for Medicaid is appropriate to help cover costs. If it is needed, they arrange for respite care. They also evaluate the insurance some families have that will pay for caregivers. They can help you find out about that being available.

Spiritual Chaplains (SCs) give the spiritual and emotional support that the patient, family, or caregiver requests. They guide individuals through spiritual and existential questions related to death. They know about significant religious and cultural rituals and routines. Religion and prayers for all denominations can be provided, but patients and families are never pushed to do so. If you are not associated with a religion, don't think you have spiritual things to talk about, or don't think you have grief issues, you can decline their services, but we strongly advise that you meet with them to really find that out. If you have nontraditional spiritual beliefs, don't assume that an SC doesn't know about them. They are trained multiculturally to offer respect to you and your rituals. They are not limited in the scope of how they can support you and your family. With no medical or financial aspects to work on, SCs can sit with the patient or family to provide whatever kind of spiritual and social support is needed.

Both the MSW and SC set a schedule for visits depending on the request of the patient or family. They can visit monthly or weekly, as is often the case, when needs change.

MD can stand for **Medical Doctor** or for hospice **Medical Director**. The MD has a full-time job in their expressed field. They are available for the nurse by phone every day to assess qualifications for admissions and recertifications, determine the medications needed, discuss symptom changes, and get new medications or treatments ordered. All team members come to team meetings every other week. The MD assesses criteria for continuing in hospice during each certification period. He or she signs official documents, educates parties on medications and treatments as needed and collaborates with the team, discussing the needs of the patients and the team. After the first six months, the nurse practitioner or MD will come to visit. That assessment is to ensure that the patient is showing some decline and continues to need hospice services.

Nurse Practitioners (NPs) provide palliative care services for all home health patients and consult with the MD and RN/CM in hospice agencies. They make visits to the hospital, SNF, or home to see a patient who has a particularly difficult symptom to manage. This is usually at the request of the RN/CM and nursing supervisor who need additional assessments done to determine the best treatment. State requirements exist for NPs working under the supervision of an MD. An NP can write orders and educate the patient, family, or staff about those changes. After the first six months, the NP or MD will come to visit. That assessment is to ensure that the patient is showing some decline and continues to need hospice services.

If NPs become involved, they co-manage the patient with the RN/CM. They are often the wound-care specialists in an agency. Many patients don't ever have the need to see the NP, but this is a great resource to have. NP education requires having a masters degree in a particular area of nursing practice.

Nursing Supervisor is the clinical director of all the staff on the hospice team. This role requires the person to be an RN, usually with a masters degree and several years of experience in hospice care, who manages the administrative needs of the team. They monitor all the care given to the patients; interview, hire, train, and supervise clinical staff; collaborate at the team meetings; and work to maintain the agency's status with state and federal agencies.

Volunteers receive special training to know about grieving. Unlike the SC or MSW, they can just be present to visit patients in hospitals, SNFs, or homes as another social contact for the patient. Many patients request or need to talk with someone about favorite things because they have no local family. Hospice agencies try to provide that extra person who has no other obligation to the patient than to be there for them and enjoy some time together, so the patient then knows that someone cares about them and will gladly make weekly visits to be with them.

Marketing Staff are critical to hospice care. They are the ones who initiate and maintain a relationship with all the medical and ancillary staff whose professions are represented in all the hospitals and SNFs. Without their skill in promoting the agency, we wouldn't have the patients, and the agency would not survive. They visit hospitals, doctor's offices, facilities that care for handicapped children and adults, places where seniors choose to live, assisted living facilities, and independent living facilities. They keep up to date on all the regulations for CMS and insurance companies and know every aspect of hospice. As such, they often do meet and greets, get consents signed, and order equipment. They often are the first person to show the patient and family about this program that really cares about all members of the family during this difficult time.

Vigil Services include persons who may or may not be CNAs. They are requested by families who cannot be there to sit at the bedside of a patient when death becomes imminent. Many people are concerned that someone should not die alone. This is not a CMS-supported service, so vigil staff are available from some agencies that are large and well supported by donors. If the staff person is not also a CNA, they cannot do the personal care, and the family must provide that. The vigil staff do observe the patient and report to the RN/CM as needed, hold the person's hands, play music, speak to them, and often are a fabulous calming presence during a person's last days and hours.

Complementary Care is that given by massage therapists, Reiki and Healing Touch practitioners, and music therapists, which are available in some larger agencies. This is not a CMS-supported service, but we wish it was. Some agencies pay these staff, and other agencies have volunteer staff providing this remarkable care. Complementary care can be critically helpful in reducing anxiety, agitation, and pain symptoms. There actually is a music degree for assisting in hospice care, and harpists and other stringed-instrument musicians have been critically important for being at the bedside for hours and often for the actual death of patients.

Bereavement Services (also known as grief counseling) is done by the MSW and SC staff who are available to counsel and support families after the death has occurred. Some families need this support right away; for others, it starts several weeks after the death; and for some, none is needed. Regardless, it is available for 13 months after the patient's death. The bereavement staff may not be the same MSW or SC that was with the patient and family prior to the death.

Pharmacy Services include specialized pharmacies that may have routine business as well. These are not chains like CVS or Walgreens, but they may be small neighborhood pharmacy businesses. They keep hospice's required medications in stock while others do not, and they routinely deliver them the same day, up to about 10 p.m., and have on-call drivers for the rare emergencies requiring a delivery throughout the night. This system is in place to ensure that patients get the medications they need as soon as possible. They have the capability of compounding common or unusual combinations of drugs found to alleviate symptoms without using injections. Those medications are not carried by regular pharmacies, and many doctors don't even know about them. Someday, every doctor will have hospice patients and learn about the aggressive use of medications that can be given without adding pain.

Durable Medical Equipment refers to companies that provide hospital beds, side rails, wheelchairs, tables, shower chairs, commodes, and respiratory equipment like nebulizers and oxygen concentrators. They deliver these items to the home and maintain the supplies and repairs.

Medical Supply Companies, such as McKesson, Apria, or Medline, will deliver pull-up and tabbed briefs, gloves, lotion, bathing supplies, creams, wound supplies and much more. The staff assesses the need for refills early in the week to try to prevent a patient from running out on a weekend. The companies only take orders from the agency staff. Families are encouraged to call the agency if there is a shortage of supplies.

Coroner Services are a required contact in some counties when a patient starts hospice care. They are contacted again at the time of death prior to reaching out to a funeral home or crematory. Some other counties allow the funeral home or crematorium to report the date, time, and cause of death, as stated by the hospice staff attending the patient.

For Emergencies or After-Hours Calls for Help

At the start of care, every family is informed that they should not call 911 and that they need to have the Do Not Resuscitate (DNR) paper handy in case someone mistakenly does dial 911. The worst-case scenario is that the ambulance arrives, the patient has stopped breathing, and those in attendance cannot produce the DNR. For a frail elderly patient to undergo CPR, which the EMTs are required to do in that circumstance, is brutal! Ribs can be broken, and since the death was not unexpected, a new tragedy has just occurred. Make sure that the DNR is situated in a very conspicuous location and that you tell all visitors you do not want them to call 911.

Rare instances occur with a fall that results in a non-life-threatening fracture and/or a condition totally unrelated to the hospice diagnosis. Then a trip to the ER is needed. All families and facility staff are instructed to call the hospice agency right away for anything if they even consider that emergency help is needed. The hospice agency will help determine what the need is; in many instances it is not a hospital trip. For emergency care not related to hospice, calling the agency is still necessary to arrange for hospice to be stopped temporarily, so they are not billed for the care being received. Hospice will be restarted upon the person's return home.

Calling the agency any time of the day or night will get you information on how to manage a change in symptoms or the death of the patient. The on-call nurse and the scheduled night shift triage nurse can see on the computer everything about the patient. By knowing what the diagnosis, medications, and treatments are, they can make a recommendation to deal with the new symptom. They will determine whether sending a nurse is the best idea. If a nurse visit is not needed, they will follow up with you by phone 30–45 minutes later to see how the patient has responded to the treatment and how you are doing. They also will notify the team, and that follow-up will happen in the morning.

Pronouncement Process

When death happens for hospice patients, do not call 911. Hospice agencies have been given full authority to declare a death if that person was under their care. The family contacts the agency when they determine that the breathing and pulse have ceased for a few minutes. The agency assigns a staff member—registered nurse, medical social work, or spiritual chaplain—to come and pronounce that the patient has died. To assist the family, they will call the funeral home or crematorium or make calls to relatives, as requested. They call the coroner, as applicable. They will stay with the family to offer support and will not leave until the deceased has been removed from the house and is safely in the transporting vehicle. These professionals will stay with the family longer if there is a need for more support or counseling.

Chapter 3:
The Physical, Psychological, Emotional, Spiritual, and Metaphysical Changes of Decline

Certain patterns of decline are seen in the kinds of illnesses that lead to death. In this chapter, I use stories from actual experiences with patients to describe a few of the physical, mental, spiritual, and metaphysical changes that are common. These changes herald that specific point on the trajectory where health dramatically angles down. This may help both patients and family members become more prepared.

Three major trajectories are shown in Figure 1 to provide a visual image of the disease patterns referred to in this chapter. The descriptive names are Short, Intermediate with Acute Episodes, and Gradual Dwindling Physical and Cognitive Frailty.

1. **Short:** This describes cancer, which includes pancreatic, lung, and colon. Patients have high function for a while and then have a sudden decline in function, which requires complete care for a while.

2. **Intermediate with Acute Episodes:** This describes organ failure and includes liver disease, chronic lung and heart conditions, kidney failure, and stroke. These patients experience a decline that consists of intermittent crises and then some improvements or plateaus. Death might occur without warning from a heart attack or stroke. This group has the most unpredictable timeframe.

3. **Gradual Dwindling Physical and Cognitive Frailty:** This can include Alzheimer's disease and other forms of dementia, Parkinson's disease, or ALS, in which much of the patient's function is lost in the early years of their disease and then they need convalescent supportive care for long periods of time.

Figure 1. Trajectory of Decline for Hospice Patients

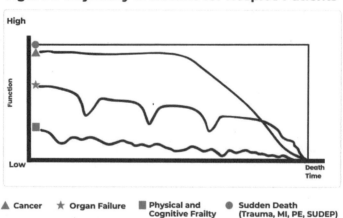

Adapted from Illness Trajectories and Palliative Care

Note: In Figure 1, the top trajectory refers to Sudden Death.
(The list includes trauma, myocardial infarction, pulmonary
embolism, and SUDEP, which stands for Sudden Death in
Epilepsy.)

Many short pamphlets or fliers have been prepared for families
and handed out as they enter hospice care that usually include
a similar graph with a timeframe and lists of symptoms
common for most patients as they progress through the "dying
process." Those lists include physical, emotional, spiritual, and
metaphysical changes.

Physical Changes

The physical changes that happen to most people are:

- Decreased appetite
- Weight changes
- Muscle weakness
- Infections
- Increased fatigue and
  sleeping
- Dehydration
- Incontinence
- Constipation
- Nausea and vomiting
- Wounds
- Immobility
- Blood pressure changes
- Body temperature changes
- Labored breathing
- Clammy skin
- Glassy eyes
- Apnea
- Gurgling
- Mottled skin

Unless there is a sudden death, the last of these from "blood
pressure changes" on usually occur in the last few days to hours
of a person's life. The first 11 cover many symptoms that may
happen early in the course of disease or may never happen at

all. These are explained in more detail in Chapter 6.

The stages of decline depend on far too many factors to give a precise timeline. In the pamphlets and fliers, the authors make sure to point out the many exceptions to the time estimates. Most people go through these changes, but not everyone does. Trying to set the timeframe for those to occur (as in months, weeks, days, and hours) before death also can be misleading. If someone changes dramatically outside the boundaries of those charts or tables, the patient or family often fear they will die that much sooner, which may not be the case as with the information about UTI that follows. On the other hand, sudden changes also can herald a shorter timeframe. The rest of this section offers stories that may help prepare families and caregivers.

Complexity of a Urinary Tract Infection (UTI)

This is an example of something that can happen to anyone, not just dementia patients, to throw time predictions out the window. Around 60% of people with dementia die either from a bladder infection or UTI that becomes septic or a lung infection. The progression from the onset of that infection to death due to sepsis can happen to anyone and occur in as short as 48 hours.

A UTI is the most common type of infection, so the following is how that progression often goes from infection to sepsis (which is an overwhelmed immune system) to death.

Patients often lose the ability to properly empty their bladder, and many wear pull-up briefs for a long time, so bacteria are always present on the skin. When urine remains in the bladder because of incomplete emptying and the patient doesn't get cleaned carefully, a bladder infection can happen. A common symptom in patients who lack body awareness is that they may not feel any pain when they urinate. In that circumstance, family and staff might not know of discomfort until major changes occur in the patient's condition.

If the infection isn't treated in time, a person may become septic. That can mean that the infection is in the bloodstream and spreading to all the organs and tissues, overwhelming the organs, and possibly leading to death. Many people can survive sepsis if their immune system is strong and they get the right medications soon enough.

A signal that the body is overwhelmed is when all the organs start shutting down. If a person is at the hospital and not in hospice, the staff will do blood tests frequently and be able to see changes indicating that the liver, heart, and kidneys are shutting down. Thus, they may be able to do something about the symptoms.

In the home or a nursing home, a hospice patient does not get any tests that require needles, so blood draws are not done. Even without machines and tests, one can tell from the urine output how the kidneys are doing. They can assess the person's color from head to foot and know whether the heart and circulatory system are shutting down. They can know from speaking to the patient about their cognitive status, and, while doing turns and personal care in the bed, they can know about their muscle strength and independence of movement.

When septic, it may only take 48 hours for a patient's organs to completely shut down and result in death. In most instances, it happens so fast that people die with no apparent pain. Pain and anxiety medications are available and used both in facilities and in the homes of the patients, if needed.

Sudden changes with a bladder infection include confusion; being delusional or hallucinating; the loss of balance and strength, which may result in falls; or decreased appetite and thirst that leads to dehydration. Of course, which came first, dehydration or the infection?

The correct antibiotic usually will resolve all of this in 7–14 days, but if the person has no fever, doesn't complain of pain, and wears a brief, no one knows whether they have an increased frequency of urination, which is another sign.

So how can we tell if they are infected? Another symptom to watch out for is the color and smell of the urine. If they wear briefs, there will be a brownish color and the strong odor of infected urine. Once detected, did the infection get treated in time or was it too late? Only time will tell.

This example brings up a very important and not uncommon reality about hospice care. Antibiotics may delay a person's death, but they will not prevent it.

Fact: A person is in hospice because they have a terminal illness.

Fact: Many people have repeated infections from which they have recovered due to antibiotics, but they never recover to the full functionality they had before.

Fact: Each body dies from one or another medical problem that overwhelms their ability to have a life of quality as they define it.

Fact: Repeated infections can be construed as the way that this particular body is presenting what the cause of death most likely will be. In other words, this body is telling everyone what the exit strategy (cause of death) might be.

With repeated infections, the hospice staff will ask the family whether it is best to treat what is expected to happen in the future. If the patient has symptoms of pain, absolutely treatments are given. With no symptoms of pain, which is the case with most sepsis patients, consider whether there is a benefit to treating it or whether the person's body should be allowed to finish what it started and permit the ending that seems to be desired. This is what I call a "tough love" situation in hospice!

Another lesson I learned through the years was that many patients with this constellation of symptoms were being admitted to hospice only to find out that the person was not near death. Many people recover close to their functionality they had before the infection. Some hospice programs will continue services for the first 90 days, which concludes the first certification period, but when the person recovers sufficiently, they must be discharged from hospice even if it is sooner than the 90 days.

CMS is quite strict about patients meeting the criteria for admission as well as meeting criteria during the full certification period. These rules have taught most hospice programs to wait at least 14 days after diagnosis and treatment of a UTI to know whether hospice is the correct direction for care of the patient.

Clinical Scenarios

The following stories reveal trajectory changes that required major shifts in care. They cover two of the trajectories and involve multiple categories of anticipated changes.

- The tumor moves to a critical place, eliminating one or more organ functions.
- The brain tumor mimics neurological diseases that affect the spine and brain at a new and critical place, eliminating physical and organ functions.

Cancer and Organ Failure: A woman had lung cancer, and her tumor was on the edge of one lung that was close to the esophagus (tube to the stomach). It grew just a little bit larger, which made all the difference in the world! In addition to affecting more lung tissue, it literally pushed up against the esophagus. This issue was critical because she suddenly had intractable nausea from the pressure and less lung tissue for breathing.

While oxygen-dependent, she previously had been ambulatory and taking care of herself within her home. Then, all in one day, she became so weak from the lack of oxygen and inability to eat that she needed medication for her intolerable nausea, a hospital bed to be brought in, and someone to take care of her. I was there for about 10 hours that first day and evening on the phone with the hospice doctor and pharmacy and using medications from the comfort kit then getting other medications delivered. We tried three different ones before getting control of her nausea and vomiting. I called her friend over, and she observed and learned about the administration of medications and all the care. Another terrific friend came over the next day to share in the caregiving.

The tumor growth moved so fast that she was gone in just three short days. She never got out of bed again, she stopped eating and drinking, and her spirit said, "It's time to move on." The fight to stay alive was traded for an acceptance of death, and she transitioned comfortably because she was cared for by trusted friends, she was ready, and she was made comfortable with the right medications.

Cancer Can Mimic a Neurological Disease: When a tumor grows, more neurons are suddenly affected as with Parkinson's disease or a stroke. When that happens, suddenly the body loses more physical function: muscle weakness, reduced coordination, cognitive changes, altered communication ability (speaking or understanding), eating ability, and incontinence—all in 48 hours.

The younger the person is, the harder it will be to convince them that they must call for assistance before trying to move about. For a 40-year-old with a brain tumor, giving up independence in any of the activities of daily living is a huge blow to their dignity. It took three falls within two days to convince one man that the side rails of his bed were not for climbing over like when he was 6 years old. They were a physical barrier to detain him for his safety and to remind him to call for help. When the family provided full-time care, he had their help and assurance that he was loved and cared for despite being less physically capable. This could be the situation for someone with COPD or heart disease, too. Anyone can be ambulatory and somewhat independent one day and then bedbound and dependent the next.

Psychological, Emotional, Spiritual, and Metaphysical Changes and Experiences

Following are examples of the psychological, emotional, and spiritual issues and changes that may happen in the months, weeks, or days before death:

- Threatened ego
- Fear
- Feelings of losing control
- Shock or denial
- Anger
- Bargaining
- Concerns about essence, meaning, and purpose
- Legacy concerns
- Predeath anxiety

Any of these issues can happen long before the decline and
then show up again near death. One can imagine from the
previous story—about the 40-year-old who fell three times and
had some of these issues—that it helps when the family and
caregivers know about these changes so they can help the
patient grieve those losses. It also helps caregivers be more
aware for anticipating their own grief.

Predeath Anxiety

Predeath anxiety occurs in many patients and describes their
unique and needy behavior that perhaps heralds the need to
spend more time and bring in everyone who needs to say their
"closure" comments to the patient. Although the patient may
have no other physical dying symptoms, the patient becomes
needy for attention and companionship. Most of the time
when this neediness occurs, it is a signal that death is only a
few weeks away.

The word "anxiety" in this label can be misleading because the
patient is often very calm and sure about what they want or
need. One very clear thing to families and caregivers is that the
patient requests and complains about things that are real, but
the expression of those needs follow one right after the other.
They are accompanied by comments like "I'm so glad to see
you" or "Come sit with me a minute" or "Do you have to go?"
The family or caregiver thinks, "I was just in there and we did
that already."

It soon becomes clear that the patient does not want to be alone. They also need reassurance that, on some level, they are aware that their leaving is really happening and that they need to know that everyone will be okay after they leave. A parent doesn't want to burden a child and vice versa, but they don't quite know how to ask those validating questions, so it shows in their requests for time and taking care of details.

This doesn't necessarily mean that the patient needs someone continuously present with them, but they are asking for someone to be with them more than before. This change may only be for a few hours or days, but the family and caregivers do need to change the schedule.

When this phase is complete, the patient knows that they can let go. The family comes together, so they are present to talk about everything and anything that gives the patient pleasure about the life they lived. This is a good time to bring in relatives or best friends from across the state or the country.

This also is a time when the staff members will inform families that, if they haven't done so yet, it's the time to say, "It's okay to go," or offer validating comments about how great your relationship was as a spouse, child, or extended family. They need to know that you will miss them, but that you will be okay when they're gone. You can talk about what their "legacy" will look like.

In the last days, hours, or minutes, you might notice any of the
following in patients:

- Turning within
- Increased contemplation
- Clouding of consciousness
- Confusion
- Delirium
- Coma
- Enhanced clarity
- Depression
- Grief
- Sorrow
- Guilt
- Regret
- Anxiety
- Helplessness
- Hope
- Anxiousness
- Acceptance
- Needing permission to die
- Visions and talking about their communication with
  others not visible or audible to anyone else
- Sense of preparing to travel or take a journey
- Sense of expectancy
- Metaphysical experiences

Many of these occurrences fall into the category of "predeath
anxiety" or perhaps "predeath expectancy!"

Metaphysical Experiences

In the last 20 years, many more people have come to know and accept having metaphysical experiences. These occurrences can happen weeks before death, and the patient may talk freely about them. This is one of the absolute joys I've experienced with patients and families. Their opportunity to share with the rest of us what it's like to be straddling two worlds and speak about what they see and feel is a treasure, gift, and confirmation to many that there is an afterlife that is peaceful and something to anticipate.

Previously, many families and doctors thought people were delusional and needed to take psychotropic drugs to control those thoughts. Unless someone is so agitated and anxious that they cannot relax and are demonstrably afraid of what they are seeing and talking about, medications are not used.

However, if you, the family, or caregiver, express denial or disagreement with what they say, that agitation might just be their way of telling you that you have suddenly become the enemy! Losing trust in the caregivers is what is at stake. If the patient thinks anyone doubts that their experiences are not possible or true or valid or anyone disagrees with them, the patient may very well begin to fear everyone and no longer take medicine or food and fight all aspects of their care.

Whether those caring for the patient believe in an afterlife or that predeceased loved ones can be present from another dimension is not the critical piece. The patient is telling us that they believe it, and they need to have that validated without question. The patient needs to know they are safe while making this transition and that they are correct in whatever they tell us they are seeing and hearing and feeling. They can discuss what they see because they have moved into this new metaphysical dimension or reality or phase of the transition.

Caregivers are all advised to have a discussion with the patient and never say or infer that it's a delusion or imagination or a dream unless they use those words themselves. Be with them in this new state of their reality and learn as much as you can about it! This is the perfect time to ask them who they see, where they are, or what they are being told or asked to do. Our curiosity validates this for them, and we get to learn more about what the dying experience can be.

If they think there are being visited by their mother or Jesus or a Native American chieftain and/or they say they're going to die by the weekend, it's imperative that you do not disagree with them. Find a way to support, acknowledge, do, and say anything to show them that you believe them—no matter how hard it is—in order to maintain the relationship of trusted caregiver. Pain medicine might still be needed, and, if the patient no longer trusts you, they will fight you like you are their worst enemy and think you are poisoning them. Then they might end up with physical—and certainly mental—suffering that is unnecessary.

Clinical Scenarios

The following stories predominantly involve psychological, emotional, spiritual, and metaphysical experiences. Some of them show how patients see beyond this life. One story describes a doctor's resistance to hospice care while the last two demonstrate how critical it is for family members to have what it takes to do the care for their family member.

Validation Denied: A family had three sons with a dying mother. One son was not present when this phenomenon was first explained by the nurse, but he was the one present when the patient first talked about seeing her husband sitting on a park bench, wearing his golf clothes and a red hat, and telling her to join him. The son didn't believe in this metaphysical possibility and told her that it could not have happened.

When I arrived that morning, she complained to me about that son, saying she refused to eat what he served her because she suspected that the food was poisoned. This is a common response in this type of situation. She clearly demonstrated her sudden fear of him. Then she told me about what she had seen. She called it a dream and that it had happened three nights in a row. She asked me if it was possible. Using her words, I said that it was a delightful dream, and that was a very common experience for patients like her. I added that I hoped she would feel safe to go with him the next time it happened.

I took time in another room to engage the help of the other sons because of the one's reluctance and ignorance about this dynamic. They were able to explain it to him so he understood, and he agreed to try talking with her. Thankfully, he succeeded. This situation made a believer out of him. All it took was him explaining that he now remembered his dad's favorite red golfing hat, and he calmly apologized for doubting her. His mother immediately calmed down and smiled, and they all talked about their father a while longer. She loved her sons and finally felt accepted by all of them. During the remainder of the day, she accepted food, care, and her pain medications. We have to assume that she went with her husband that night after getting the validation she needed from her sons.

Validation Given: When the chaplain meets a patient, one of the topics raised is whether they have any association with any specific religious community. One patient said that he was a very active Jehovah's Witness. He was from Mexico, was bilingual, and was living with his daughter's family. Because we know of the phenomenon in which people close to dying see and talk to others, we all eventually speak with our patients about that. He was asked about the church's beliefs about an afterlife, and the patient said that they believe that death is the end of one's life, that there is no reincarnation, and nothing happens after death. They believe that people have only one life, and that's it. He never believed that loved ones come to talk with people who are dying.

Well, you can already imagine where this is going. One day, a few months later, he spoke to me about seeing and talking to his mother. I brought his daughter into the room because, in case she didn't know, I wanted her to validate for him that this was fine and wonderful and to tell us all about it. I asked him how he felt about that, knowing that his religion taught him it was not possible. He very calmly said, "They're wrong. I know my mother. She comes to talk to me, and I see her as well."

One day a teenage grandson was walking down the hallway and overheard his grandfather speaking. He stepped into the room and asked him about it, and the patient very calmly reported to him about the conversation he was having with his mother who was sitting next to him at the side of the bed with her arm around him. The grandson told his family that there was no one else physically in the room. Everyone was fine knowing about this, and it led up to an amazing dying moment. He later actually announced that he knew when he was going to go be with his mother! With his family sitting in his room as he was lying in bed, he raised his arm up and over, held it there as if he were hugging someone, then took his last breath.

We don't often get the chance to have conversations like this that help validate these occurrences for patients. But I've had several, and some people do not act shocked after growing up being told it could not happen. It's so real for them that all they want to do is keep doing it. They feel the love from a visitor on "the other side," whatever that is, and it's our job to convey total acceptance so they approach their transition in peace. Others who are surprised will, in a hesitating voice, report on the occurrences, and many will ask permission to know that these occurrences are indeed normal. We tell them what we believe is happening, so they feel safe.

Dying Alone: At the actual end stage of knowing that death is close, the family and caregivers need to decide how to schedule their time. The idea of establishing a "vigil" is one that depends on the family's close relationship with the patient, knowing that previously in their life, they never felt secure being alone.

Statistics reveal that 85% of patients die alone. In fact, despite a vigil organized so carefully that there was not one minute where someone wasn't scheduled to be present, many patients have used the brief "I'm just going for a potty break, I promise. I won't be gone but a minute or two" time period to take their last breath and demonstrate that the person's spirit was in charge. It's hard to know the intention until that moment! This very scenario happened in a family of engineers. The sons had a schedule in an Excel spreadsheet; the patient's wife did not feel it was necessary. In addition to the question of whether a vigil is needed, this is a great example of a spouse knowing the needs of her husband but allowing the needs of the family to be satisfied.

Knowing Oneself and Being in Control: Here is an example of a patient knowing themselves well, having a strong connection to their spirit, receiving the serenity of knowing they are in control.

A 78-year-old woman, living alone, had heart disease and started needing more and more oxygen as she got weaker. She had five sons, some of whom lived only blocks away, and they took turns coming by twice a day to see that she had everything she needed. They got her meals, but she was ambulatory and able to toilet herself. She was continent and made it very clear that she would never live in a diaper. Maintaining her dignity about this physical condition was what mattered to her the most.

Her physical condition did finally deteriorate, and she became incontinent of urine... ONCE! She died sometime during the night, hours after her son had to help her to the bathroom and aid with her hygiene. Her son came by at his usual time in the morning to help her with breakfast and found her comfortably in her bed, no longer alive.

A Doctor's Hubris: This story is about the patient's choice to stop treatment and what happened when her doctor objected. It is a sad example of a doctor's hubris. This mentality was already rare by 2016, but it did happen.

An oncologist challenged me and the family of the patient in my care by telling us that only he, not the nurses, could tell if a person was dying, and he was recommending more chemo. He refused to accept that this patient was alert and verbal and decisional 48 hours before when she needed hospitalization for symptoms related to her cancer.

After being admitted to the hospital, she asked the family to stop the treatments, so the hospital staff contacted our hospice. Together with her family, they talked with her about what that entailed, and she accepted. Everyone agreed that they didn't want her to suffer any longer, so the focus changed to hospice care, which would allow her to be more comfortable until she transitioned. Since she was in the hospital for a medical crisis related to her cancer and was too fragile to be sent home, even by ambulance, her billing status was changed to Medicare Hospice and she remained in the same room. To make the room quiet, the monitor was removed. To make her more comfortable, her IV was taken out, and even the pulse oxygen monitor on her finger was removed.

All her doctors were informed, but this doctor came to the room to voice his objection. One of the nurses was sharp enough to ask him to remain in the hall while she came into the room to inform me and the family about his objection and that he was in the hall wanting to talk to the family. We all went out to speak with him. He didn't believe me or the family about her status and that it was her decision to stop chemo and enter hospice. The family was enraged and told him to leave them alone and not come back. They did not allow him to enter the room to see her! She actually died the next day.

Thankfully, very few doctors treat families or nurses this way any longer. Most doctors know their patients better and they have learned to trust the hospice team's assessments of a patient's status.

The last two stories are about the families—one that could not do the necessary care and another that rose to the occasion when they thought they did not have the ability to do the required care.

Family Unable to Do the Necessary Care: This sad story relates the devastating effects of a wound and also acknowledges a significant difficulty about being a caregiver.

A bedridden patient's family was afraid to move her because it might cause her pain. Because of the lack of turns to relieve pressure and facilitate getting oxygen to her thin skin over the sacrum, the patient developed a very deep, painful wound.

The only medication that relieved the pain was morphine, but even though the team had educated the family about the function of morphine, the family feared giving it because they thought their mother would die soon afterward. This vicious cycle ended up causing everything they had feared. The adult children made promises to the staff about giving medications and doing her turns, but they just couldn't do it.

On the patient's last day, I arrived and assessed that the patient needed to be medicated. When she expressed the relief of pain, she was turned. Three family members were cowering in the kitchen, so they wouldn't have to see me give her morphine and turn her or potentially hear their mother if she groaned.

The patient was still verbal and able to smile, so her death did not appear to be imminent. She did let out a sigh, not a groan of pain, when she was moved. She then gave me a huge smile, acknowledging that she had needed that, and she fell asleep very quickly.

I knew that I had to be firmer with her children about giving her morphine and turning her from side to side only to try to prevent the pain. Of course, they were scared and sad and apologetic. I understood their reluctance, knowing they never wanted to hurt her. I even contacted the social worker and spiritual counselor to possibly intervene as well. I let them know that I'd be back in the morning, but the patient did what many others have done before her. She assessed her physical condition as being ready to die peacefully and relieved her children of the dreaded tasks of taking care of her.

The timing was the big surprise. Just 15 minutes after I left—I was still in the car on the way to another patient—the call came in. I turned around smiling, knowing that she had finally been comfortable enough to let go.

This is a good example for two reasons. It's about how difficult it is for a person to let go and die if they are uncomfortable. It also is about the difficulty some people have being a caregiver. The instructions for administering medications are carefully determined to ensure the patient's comfort. If a family member cannot handle their own grief and emotions when temporarily causing discomfort, the hard truth is that they need to hire someone else who can emotionally handle this kind of stress. A personally detached caregiver can make or break a good hospice situation.

All families need to know themselves well enough to decide who among them should or should not give personal care. Tell the other members to fill the medication box, make meals, or pay the bills. They can still be involved, but they can do something comfortable for them.

The assessments done by the registered nurse, social worker, and spiritual chaplain should be able to figure this out. It often seems like everything will be fine in the beginning. Parents and children never want to burden each other, but when it becomes apparent that there are serious challenges to the patient getting the necessary care, we suggest hiring someone or transferring the patient to a facility where the family members can visit and not see or hear what disturbs them so much.

Unprepared Family Rises to the Occasion: This story is about a family learning lessons about themselves. In this instance, the patient did not suffer because of any lack of care. It is an amazing example of a person staying alive waiting for a social and spiritual event to occur.

I admitted a woman to hospice who was dependent on a walker and lived alone. I don't even remember her diagnosis because that was not the important part of this learning experience. Her three sons and their wives were present during the admission, but they strangely stayed in the living room instead of joining their mother and me. At the end of the admission process, she suddenly laid back onto the bed with her eyes closed, and she did not respond to questions or physical touch. She most likely had a stroke because she was unconscious and only breathing three times a minute.

I reported to my boss and then to the family to begin teaching them about the 24/7 care they were going to have to manage starting right then! Of course, they were all shocked. But what surprised me was that they argued with each other about who would be able to do all of it because each one said they could not and pleaded with the others to take charge! They eventually got quiet, so I could show them how to do the direct care. I was able to provide them with some briefs and tell them what to get at the store until the next day when the supply order would arrive. I gave instructions about the comfort kit and symptoms to watch for, how to give medications, and when to call the office, fully expecting that she would die that night. Eventually I left their home.

For the next three days, I returned each morning to find her alive but still breathing only three times per minute. Each day some of her children were present, and each day they argued less and cooperated more. On Day 3, she died. They all were following their schedule to fully take care of her, and they made the funeral arrangements. It appeared to me that she survived long enough for her family to come together and work as a team.

Knowing what to anticipate and how to comfort and protect the patient physically, emotionally, and spiritually helps the staff prepare the families and caregivers to do the same. We hope to have the time to help everyone be more ready, and this book is one step toward that education.

Chapter 4:
Medication Management

Medication education is ongoing and includes helping the family and caregivers learn the names and purposes of each medication, so when the condition changes, they have a basic understanding of whether those changes are related to the medication or not.

The family or hired caregiver is required to administer all the medications. A list is written out, and whatever is needed (such as lists in other languages) is provided. Initially, this may be no different than the management to which the family was accustomed. As changes are made, the nurse ensures that the family and caregiver know what to give, why, and how. As symptoms change, the family must know whether to notify the agency right away or if they can wait until the next nurse's visit to get instructions on what to do, if they need that.

Hospice medications generally do not include injections or IV fluids. It is decided on a case-by-case basis. The principle behind this is to avoid doing any procedure that is invasive and painful, which includes the administration of medications. For patients who are not in palliative care or hospice, the common frequency for giving pain medications is every 4–6 hours. In palliative care and hospice, we evaluate patient responses and watch and listen to learn how frequently their pain returns. If the patient is able, we ask them for a rating and teach everyone involved that on a scale of 1–10, the 1–3 is considered managed. A verbal or visual rating, with caregivers estimating the grimaces, at 4–6 is considered unmanaged and time to repeat the dose. Ideally, we want to prevent a rating of 7–10. If their pain returns much earlier than expected, the dose and/or frequency will be changed, so it is controlled. Controlling pain and all other symptoms is the top priority for all hospice staff.

Shortness of breath is another symptom that shows variations that require medication and/or dose changes and are evaluated all day, every day. Counting the number of breaths per minute and watching the patient's face and chest to see how labored they appear is taught to patients and families as well. We do that so the patient can move, eat, socialize, and sleep to their satisfaction—in other words "have a life!"

This is where the phrase "quality of life" that you see in the literature about hospice care programs comes in. Establishing symptom management to the level that the patient reports it as controlled allows them the comfort to be less stressed and more able to do whatever they're capable of doing in their life that they describe as their "quality of life."

On the day of admission, every patient receives a "comfort kit" or "symptom-management kit," which includes several medications typically used to manage end-of-life symptoms. This kit that comes from the pharmacy includes a sheet of paper explaining each medication, and the admission nurse reviews that with the family and caregivers, so they have a basic knowledge of what to give when, why, and how. The hospice staff does not expect laypersons to memorize all that information, but it is the nurse's job to review it with them before leaving them to care for their loved ones.

The nurse provides a written list with all the medications, not just the comfort kit meds. Special medications are provided on Day 1 because of the phenomenon of sudden changes in their condition that sometimes happen upon hospice admission. Many times, when the patient has a sense that "everyone feels safe now so I can go," the patient chooses to transition that same day without going through all the typical changes that could occur from their terminal diagnosis. Some may need a few doses of some of those medications on Day 1, so that is why those medications and the education are provided.

Medications Change

Some people are under the impression that all medications taken prior to hospice are discontinued when hospice starts. That is not accurate. As presented in the Introduction section on myths, some medications may be discontinued but certainly not all of them. Medications that are no longer necessary, such as statins for reducing cholesterol, can be discontinued; and some medications given by mouth cannot be continued if a patient can no longer swallow. Every medication is identified and evaluated based on the terminal diagnosis.

A terminal diagnosis is the disease process believed to be responsible for the anticipated death within six months. Some medications taken to treat the terminal diagnosis are continued, but some may not be. If a drug is considered curative, it will be stopped because the patient and family have elected to stop curative treatments and get comfort care.

Many doctors are not trained in nutrition and do not pay attention to vitamin and mineral supplements being of value to patients and families. The nurse will discuss with the family as well as their primary care physician and hospice medical director about their use. No one can force a family to stop a medication or an over-the-counter supplement they believe has a benefit, but the family may end up needing to pay for them. The possibility of a copay for medications was presented in Chapter 2; the hospice agency decides whether a copay will be assessed and how much that will be.

Forms of Medication Delivery

Hospice care prefers to use all forms except injections or IVs for delivering medication. With patients for whom pain liquids, pills, or patches are ineffective, a method with a subcutaneous needle can be used for giving the medication. This system is commonly known as a pain med pump, which can be provided to allow the patient to remain as active as possible while being able to push a button to administer the stronger medicine on a set schedule. Different from an IV in the arm, a very short, thin needle attached to thin tubing connected to the pain pump is placed into the subcutaneous fat of the leg or abdomen. This pump can provide a continuous or scheduled infusion of pain medication. This can be used at home with the nurse visiting daily to ensure that the pain management is effective. These machines have been around a long time and are manufactured in such a way that there is a locking code that only the agency knows, so there can be no mistaken or intentional attempts to administer the narcotic medication more than scheduled.

As with all pain management, if the dose and/or frequency are not providing good management, they will be changed until proper management is achieved. Different medications might be stronger and can be tried to reduce the administration frequency so the patient and family can get more rest between the doses.

For all the other symptoms that patients experience, there are swallowable pills and liquids as well as liquids that absorb in the mouth quickly because they are highly concentrated in a small volume. Some medications are available in patches, and specialized pharmacies have created single or multidrug gels that can be rubbed on the chest or neck, all in the effort to reduce symptoms and provide comfort for hospice patients. Suppositories are also used because of the fast absorption when someone cannot take medications by mouth.

A patient's ability to swallow must be taken into account throughout their time in hospice. We must consider their physical ability as well as their alertness. Their diagnosis may prevent the ingestion of any pills. If they already have a feeding tube, which is common in patients who have had a stroke or have ALS, most medications can be crushed and put into the tube. As changes in swallowing and alertness occur, some pills can be converted into other forms. For a patient who cannot swallow, and a feeding tube is not appropriate, patches, topical creams, liquids, and suppositories must be used.

Using IVs for hydration and feeding tubes for sustenance are not used after one is admitted to hospice. Besides the fact that they can cause pain and are difficult to manage, when a person nears death, they cannot process all the extra fluids. When their appetite and thirst diminish, a person's attitude toward food is not what changes. The patient's two brains (the gastrointestinal [GI] tract and the one within the skull) actually direct those changes. When the GI system slows down its capacity to digest, it sends chemicals to the hypothalamus to slow everything down. That knob gets turned down, so they experience less hunger and thirst. That happens in partnership with the GI tract and the kidneys.

This change is not easy to notice in someone who already has a feeding tube, but there does come a time when it's necessary to stop feeding through that as well. That will be based on symptoms of the stomach digesting poorly and the kidneys reducing their function. In doing this, those organs actually protect the body from experiencing more distress. If a body does not need the nutrients, because its lifetime is nearly over, no one needs to be worried about giving food and fluids. The family is given this education early on and repeatedly. It can be especially difficult for people from some cultures for whom food is a centerpiece of their socialization. The staff hopes to educate them about this physiological functioning issue and reduce their concerns from an emotional point of view.

If the body is given more fluids than it can handle, those fluids back up, literally flooding every cell in the body. This shows up as an increase in congestion and breathing difficulty or a sudden increase in swelling everywhere from the face to the feet. Fluid in the lungs and elsewhere, which is called Third Spacing, presents an impossible complication. If a person is dying, the kidneys cannot remove that fluid, and no additional diuretic medications will make the kidneys able to do that.

Hospice does everything possible to prevent complications, not cause them. So, although the topic of IVs for giving fluids and feeding tubes is sometimes very difficult to address, we do address it, usually on the day of admission.

Controlled Substances

We do use controlled substances in hospice. Pain medications and some medications for anxiety are in that category, and the doses used to reduce symptoms are explained verbally and in writing. These explanations will be repeated as often as needed to help everyone feel comfortable about their use, expected responses, negative side effects, and when to get refills.

Quantities of medications are also assessed in the beginning of the week, so patients do not run out. Families do not call the specialized pharmacy for the refills. The pharmacies know who the agency is and will not fill any order that does not come from a nurse with that agency. Yes, even in hospice there have been instances of fraud and drug abuse by patients, their families, and staff.

Lorazepam: This is an antianxiety medication not tolerated well by some patients. Their reaction is paradoxical: They

73

become more anxious and agitated. When that happens, it is stopped, and a different medication is ordered.

Morphine: The use of morphine was addressed in the Introduction in the Dispelling Myths section, and it is covered more thoroughly with examples of the reasons people die soon after being given morphine. This is a prime example of how damaging ignorance can be. Not even pharmacists fully know about morphine until they have to use it!

Again, the terrible misconception is that morphine is used intentionally at the end of life for the purpose of ending that life! People have perpetuated this myth by thinking very superficially about the timing of its use. There have been many cases when a person has died soon after administration of morphine, but that is because that person was finally made comfortable!

It is very hard to let go when pain or breathing trouble are their dominant thoughts. When the right medication is given to achieve comfort, the patient can finally sleep, so the family needs to be prepared for the patient to pass on. This is the circumstance for most patients. One can imagine them thinking to themselves, "I'm comfortable and I'm ready and the family are all prepared. Now is a good time to go." And voilà, a person chooses to die because they physically and spiritually are able to do so.

This dynamic is explained as a possible consequence up front with the patient and their family and caregivers to reduce any fears they may have about this medication's safe and effective use.

Morphine is manufactured from a plant, which makes it organic and great for those who refuse manmade (synthetic) medications. It's the easiest and quickest pain-management medication to use.

We start with 2.5–5 mg and work up the dosage to control pain or shortness of breath by evaluating the patient every 15 minutes, not the 4- to 6-hour increments of other medications. For pain control, there is no such thing as a maximum dose! The pain receptors grab it and use it up (very quickly in some cases), so finding the right dose and frequency just takes time and paying attention!

Sleepiness and feeling groggy happens in the first 72 hours of routine use, so honor that but do not let that interfere with raising the dosage, if needed, to get control of the symptom. Some people think they have an allergy to morphine sulfate if they hallucinate or feel nauseous, but the only true allergy is anaphylaxis, during which the throat tightens and makes breathing very difficult. Other reactions are attributed to the common and mistaken administration in emergency rooms of giving too much morphine too soon via IV. With lower doses, most patients do not have those symptoms.

Other Medications: Some patients found the symptoms disturbing and simply want to know about other options. The synthetic drug Oxycodone comes in both pills and liquid form and is a great alternative. Hydromorphone appears to be a form of morphine, with the letters "morph" in it, but it isn't; its trade name is Dilaudid. This drug is actually ordered for all end-stage kidney-failure patients if they need it for breathing or pain problems because morphine can damage the kidneys. The use of other comfort kit medications is described in Chapter 5: The Dying Process.

Addiction and Overdose Concerns

When pain is managed, it means the medication is being used effectively, but if too much is given, any excess will then go to the brain and begin the process of creating addiction. As long as there is a physiological cause for pain, and medication doses are maintained, the addiction process will not happen. The medication will be soaked up where the pain exists. And please, respectfully ask yourself, "If the patient has a terminal illness, should we really be concerned about addiction?" Do not let that concern interfere with adequate symptom management.

Again, morphine or alternatives are used to treat breathing difficulties and pain. As with all medications, we start with a low dose and gradually increase it if that is needed to get control of the symptoms. We do not teach people how to use it for taking their own life. That is illegal, and we have many years of experience knowing that the orders for symptom management work for most patients.

Many countries and states have "right to die" programs that regulate how a patient can manage to take a medication or medications to facilitate their death at a time of their choosing. Since those rates vary from year to year and from state to state, this book will not document any of those statistics, but they can be easily researched. It is important to know that the legal implications of this pathway are very serious. If this subject interests you, your doctor should be the first person you ask so you can find out about all the regulations that apply to you and your loved ones in your state. You, your loved ones, and your doctor work together; each party has legal responsibilities and consequences. Having the support of your loved ones and doctors is critical to those programs because it is an enormous decision for all concerned.

Even some patients and families who asked about the "right to die" programs found that they had a very high quality of life in hospice and were able to live longer and more comfortably than they had feared.

The world of hospice medications is lightyears ahead of the ordinary use of medication. As it has been said before, you can't know everything about hospice until you've experienced it, but hopefully this book will give you the tip of its complexity iceberg.

Chapter 5:
The Dying Process

Assessing the Decline

This chapter addresses the actual physical changes that occur during the dying process. Throughout the patient's time in hospice, the nurse will pay attention to, and note, the decline in the many cognitive and physical functions to determine when a patient appears to be actively dying. Caring for a person who is dying may not be easy, but when the hospice team provides the right information to the family and caregivers, the process can be smooth.

As the patient's condition changes, the nurse will inform the family or nursing staff in facilities that the patient is "actively dying," and visits then will be done daily by the nurse. The social worker and spiritual counselor will make appointments to come right away and more often, so they can support and counsel, the certified nursing assistant may come every other day, and this also is a time for any religious organizations to send their representative for a last blessing, if that is requested.

Usually, the patient is unresponsive with their eyes closed, and they do not respond when addressed. They can hear but are unable to eat, drink, talk, make decisions, turn themselves in bed, and are incontinent of bladder and bowel. The family and/or caregivers must now check on the patient every 2–4 hours around the clock, turn them to prevent pressure sores, change their briefs, manage their bowels, provide hygiene, and administer medications as determined by the symptoms they have. If the patient shows restlessness and agitation, someone must remain with them to administer the medication and observe its effectiveness. The nurse will write down what to look for and when to give medications as well as what changes require calling the agency.

Creating a peaceful death for a patient who is actively dying is the goal. During this time, all symptoms caused by the disease progression are managed by medications or nonpharmacologic options (e.g., lavender-scented sprays, the person's favorite music, turning on a fan or opening a window, gentle massage—or ensuring that there is no massage because some patients are agitated by being touched). Energy medicine called Reiki, Healing Touch, and therapeutic music on a guitar or harp are offered by some agencies.

The patient may or may not be sedated. Some patients require medications while others move into a comatose state without sedatives. They are relaxed sufficiently to, in effect, appear to be sleeping deeply, not aware, and not affected by any of the symptoms.

This state is what I call the "Grace of the Dying Process." It is a state of being in which the patient is unaware and, therefore, not physically, emotionally, or spiritually suffering. The patient passes through this last stage, appearing to be unaware of what's going on with their body or all the care the team does.

This state is apparent when they are touched for personal care because one finds that they are like a ragdoll with completely flaccid muscles, including those in the face and jaw, and they offer no physical resistance nor verbal or nonverbal indications of discomfort. It is unknown what is actually going on in the mind of the person (who isn't talking to us), but they do not appear miserable, and the staff and family do not suffer during these hours and days until they die.

The patient's hearing is the last function to cease. Their lack of responsiveness means that it isn't possible to know what they perceive and understand; however, during this time, talking to them has the potential to provide positive, loving, grateful, and enjoyable memories. Reviewing happy times and experiences with them is strongly recommended.

Patients for whom managing symptoms is difficult exhibit obvious distress. We do have medications to reduce anxiety and agitation, and we know that it is a treatment to give those in whatever dose is required to make them less anxious or agitated. It's been a clear lesson forever that if one is suffering from pain, anxiety, agitation, fever, or difficult breathing, the spirit has a very difficult time transitioning, moving on, and letting go!

Medications are used to control symptoms that commonly occur while the body's organs gradually or suddenly shut down and cease functioning. The heart beats first in a little fetus, even before the brain and spinal cord are fully functioning, and the heart is the last organ to stop living.

During the active dying phase, the medications in the comfort kit are used. There may be some scheduled use of morphine (or its substitute), antianxiety medications, and medications that reduce excessive saliva. Other medications in the kit are used as needed. Families in the home are given a sheet of paper listing the symptoms that each medication can allay and the frequency and method of their administration. These medications are given orally, topically, or via the rectum. In skilled nursing facilities or nursing homes, these orders are also included in their computer file.

Oral medications are highly concentrated liquids, measured out in tiny quantities, to be given inside the mouth. The patient is not expected to functionally swallow. The medication absorbs quickly into the vasculature of the mouth because it's such a tiny amount. The starting dose of morphine sulfate, or a substitute liquid, is about 1/20 of a teaspoon. Knowing that anything given in the mouth generates saliva production, a few different medications are available to reduce that saliva buildup and the gurgling that accompanies it.

Even touching the inside of a person's mouth will increase the production and collection of saliva in the back of the throat. In this instance, suctioning is discouraged. The fluid settles back in the throat on the epiglottis, causing the gurgling sound with exhalation. The suction apparatus cannot be placed that far down the throat, and doing suctioning usually triggers gagging and stimulates coughing, which is distressing and thus against the hospice principle to always do whatever is possible to prevent their distress of any kind. To avoid suctioning, medications are used to dry up the excess saliva, or small sponges on a paper stick can be used to soak up the fluid.

The dying process is considered "managed" when the patient has no fever and no evident pain, nausea, vomiting, gurgling, breathing, or agitation symptoms while the organs shut down. The management is directed by the hospice nurse and the whole team, but the hour-by-hour care is done by the family, hired caregiver, or nursing home staff.

What Actually Happens When a Person Dies?

Suddenly, or gradually, the person's organs stop functioning. The lungs stop functioning and, when there is no more oxygen to feed the body, the heart stops.

Saliva Accumulation

Some think that people "choke to death," but that is not true. Even if someone has a terminal lung condition, the symptoms can be managed with oxygen and medications, so they do not appear to be struggling. Many people reported hearing fluid in the back of the throat and thought that this meant the person choked. As explained previously, there can be fluid, a small amount of saliva mixed with medications, or actual phlegm coughed up but not swallowed that remain in the throat and make a person's breathing audible. Today, it's called gurgling, but many years ago that sound was termed the "death rattle." It's a strange term, but it is factual that the description indicates that someone is near the end of life.

In addition to using medications to control that fluid buildup, it helps to turn the patient onto their side, far enough over so their face is on an angle down toward the bed. By gravity, the fluid will drain into the cheek area and away from the epiglottis. This facilitates removing the fluid with a small sponge on a paper stick. The medications used include a gel that can be rubbed on the neck or put on a patch placed behind the ear or even in drops of an oral medication, all of which can dry up saliva production. This congestion or gurgling issue is common and well known. Patients do not choke to death, and they do not appear to suffer from the gurgling.

Breathing Changes

The patient will exhibit breathing changes. For example, apnea and very fast or slow respiratory rates are a normal part of some patients' dying process. Sometimes medications will minimize this, but not always. It is important to know that we do not medicate to stop their breathing just because we know they are dying or because seeing the unusual breathing rate is uncomfortable to watch. To manage the visible signs of discomfort, gradually higher doses can be given more frequently, but it's still within the legal and physiological limits of a person's tolerance for managing symptoms.

A peaceful death does include the use of antianxiety and pain medications in safe, prescribed doses to cause a sleeping state during which death occurs. This process has been studied extensively. Hospice staff does not kill the patient nor "assist suicide." "Right to die" programs do exist, and those are presented elsewhere in this chapter.

Hospice programs follow the legalities stipulated in our licenses and in the regulations for prescribing medications, so there is no "overdosing" of medications. The doses bring the patient to a calmness that eliminates their awareness, so they have no fear, resistance, or agitation and are no longer in the "flight or fight mode" that they had before. They appear to be sleeping and that may be due to the medications used to manage symptoms that resulted in their being sedated. When patients are still in the fight or flight mode, they have trouble letting go, releasing their spirit, and dying peacefully. When we manage all the symptoms with which they are dealing, that release can happen. Having these symptoms managed well constitutes success for everyone involved.

Comfort Kit

If the comfort kit was not needed before, all those medications most likely will be needed now. Following is a list of specific symptoms and their management. Every decision about the dose and frequency of each medication must be chosen based on the needs of the patient. The generalities offered here are given in light of each nurse and doctor knowing the legalities and honoring their licenses.

- Shortness of breath and pain—liquid medication
- Anxiety and restlessness—liquid medication
- Mild pain or fever—suppository medication
- Nausea—suppository or cream
- Gurgling—cream, liquid, or patch
- Bowel movements (Constipation and impaction cause pain and discomfort.)—suppository

Again, the family and/or caregiver administer the medications unless the nurse is there when they are needed. This illustrates the critical need to have the nurse explain things well and be available to answer questions as they come up. A notepad is now required for keeping track of medication administration because that must be evaluated along with the patient's symptoms to know whether to increase a medication dosage or the frequency of when it's administered. When a patient is imminently dying or actively dying, a nurse will visit daily. The chaplain and social worker also will offer to come more often during this time to support the family and the caregivers. They also will offer to contact a minister or priest as the family desires.

What to Look for Every Few Hours and the Interventions

Pain Medications and Their Frequency: Medications are assessed at every visit and can be adjusted between visits by calling the nurse. This is critical to ensuring comfort when any kind of physical care is done. Have the nurse help you plan what that timeframe should be. Usually it is 30–60 minutes prior to doing physical care.

Pain: Grimaces and groans are indicators of pain and will be treated with the prescribed pain medications on a set schedule that all the caregivers will follow. Another principle in hospice care is to set a schedule for giving the medications when the pain rating is in the 4–6 range. This will prevent the pain from ever getting to the rating of 7–10 on the 10-point scale.

Skin: If redness, bruising, or blisters occur over any bony prominences, apply lotion, turn the patient off that area, adjust the turning frequency, and avoid any pressure to that area.

Fluid in Throat: For gurgling sounds in the throat, as described previously in detail, treat this with gel, drops in the mouth, or a 72-hour patch.

Restlessness: This presents as movements of arms, legs, and the head seemingly without purpose. This can be treated with antianxiety medications as well as medications for breathing irregularities and pain. The purposeless movements look like limbs rising then settling back down without any real action, such as scratching, changing position, or moving the sheets, being performed. To properly assess these movements, and then treat and control them, requires one to sit with the patient to observe them; these can happen every few minutes, every 15–20 minutes, or return after a few hours. Most patients do not make sounds during these, so being in another room is insufficient. The symptoms will get worse if untreated and are a sign of agitation or restlessness caused by circulation changes and nervous system discomfort. They can be as strong an interference as pain in causing distress and delaying dying.

Nausea/Vomiting: These depend greatly on the diagnosis and can be controlled by a topical gel or a rectal suppository.

Constipation: Compacted bowels can cause discomfort, so suppositories may be used as often as every three days. Especially if constipating pain medications are used, this is highly recommended.

Changes in Breathing: If breathing becomes faster, slower, or apneic, it should be treated. The eventual slowing of respirations is expected, but treating labored breathing and faster rates is essential. Maintaining a respiratory rate of 28 or fewer breaths per minute is a good target number. Most patients do not appear to be laboring at this rate. Above that number, the body heats up and creates a fever, which needs to be reduced (see Fever).

Many people want oxygen used to help breathing, but many patients already have been dependent on it, and stopping oxygen for them would never be considered. When we think of artificially keeping a person alive, we need to seriously think, in each case, about what oxygen does. The heart receives the oxygenated blood from the lungs and feeds its own muscles first. Then it fills up the ventricles and pumps to the rest of the body. This additional oxygen keeps the heart alive longer. If the lungs and heart are not diseased, room air is a natural source of oxygen for the body. If it is coming into the lungs from a machine via a nasal cannula, it's not natural.

When death is certain, all closures have happened between friends and family, and the patient is unconscious and totally dependent for every bit of care, it's common to have the "tough love" conversation with the family about whether the person would consider oxygen an artificial intervention and the life, full of quality, that they would want. For most families it's a clear choice that results in a peaceful death a little sooner. No one knows for sure how much longer a person will live on 1–1.5 liters of oxygen, but higher doses fall into this artificial category. Sometimes that's the lowest the family or facility will allow. Whatever they choose is acceptable. It is the job of the registered nurse, social worker, and spiritual chaplain to offer this different understanding; however, the family decides the right thing for that family. This is a different consideration not commonly reported, and it can be a blessing to honor someone's wishes by removing anything that is "artificial."

Morphine, or its substitute, may be used, but as stated before it does not guarantee that those breathing patterns will change. It is usually possible that it will reduce a high rate, but we are never sure which pattern is that patient's last pattern. When the breaths are very shallow, and only the upper chest and jaw move, it is called agonal breathing. The diaphragm contracts and relaxes minimally. It's obvious that the entire lung masses are not being affected by these short movements because there is almost no air exhaled. When very little air is inhaled, very little oxygen is moving through the body. Many people do not go through these various patterns; their diaphragm simply slows down and stops over time.

Circulation: Effective circulation is important. Watch the color of hands, feet, knees, and lips, which usually will turn blue or bluish/mottled. Treat this probable tingling sensation with pain medication. At this stage, the brain has directed the veins in the limbs to relax and gradually stop pushing the blood back to the heart. The brain sets the priorities and tells the limb circulation to slow to a crawl while the bulk of the oxygenated blood goes to the internal organs.

Fever: This is the body temperature. As circulation slows, the temperature of the limbs becomes cool to cold unless there is a fever warming the body and delaying the process. All families must have a thermometer because, near death, a fever usually happens from the heart and lungs' desperate attempts to feed the body and remain functional.

We treat this because it can be uncomfortable. A fever is caused by a racing heart, which causes racing respirations, and those movements increase the body's internal temperature. A racing heart rate and respiratory rate are uncomfortable, as is a fever above 100.0° F. This is a vicious, cyclical metabolic phenomenon: The body wants to stay alive, so the heart beats faster, which causes the lungs to expand and contract faster to keep up with blood flow, and that faster action inside the body creates a fever. How does the body deal naturally with a fever? It causes the lungs to expand and contract more often, and the heart beats faster to keep up! This creates a vicious cycle that causes more discomfort and perpetuates the fever. If caught early enough, giving one acetaminophen suppository together with the pain/breathing medication and antianxiety medication will reduce this metabolic fever and the discomfort it creates. Placing cool compresses in the areas with a lot of surface vasculature, like the head, armpits, groin, and feet, also is a huge help in reducing fever. If caught early, the metabolic fever only peaks once.

Ideal Medication Management: If they are needed, pain, breathing, and restlessness medications are given every 4–6 hours around the clock. The patch for oral secretions is changed every three days. It is usually possible to find the right dose to allow the caregivers and patient to have four hours of actual rest at a time in between doses. The hospice staff will explain that we rarely stop giving medications at this stage. We have had the misfortune of learning that symptoms can come back, and we don't want the patient to suffer. We have learned that it's just better to keep giving the medications to maintain the comfort we are sure about rather than risk being wrong.

Use of Machines: Even for patents in hospitals who are dying, the monitors are removed from the room. Observing the patient's skin color and the rise and fall of the chest tells the story. Many nurses still rely on a blood pressure (BP) machine and pulse oximeter, but many do not. If we see the body color become mottled, we know that the BP is very low, perhaps 60/40, and the pulse oximeter reads that the oxygen saturation is very low. When this occurs, a pulse oximeter will not be able to detect the pulse anyway. At this stage, we know that the person probably only has a few hours left, but there have been many surprises. This stage can last a few days. When asked how long the patient may live, or how soon they will die, hospice staff usually couch their answers with "maybe" and "could be" because only the person's spirit knows for sure when they will die.

Breathing Stops: When the lungs do stop, we advise waiting a few minutes more and then feeling the chest, the neck, or the wrist where it's sometimes possible to feel the heartbeat/pulse as well. For an adult, when both have stopped for about 5 minutes, it is time to call the agency. Again, never call 911. It is not uncommon for a child or teenager's heart to start beating again even 15 minutes after it has ceased beating. The will to live is an amazing thing.

Body Color Change After Death: If you are witnessing the death, you will notice a very rapid change in the person's color. With the blood no longer under the pressure of the arteries and veins to keep it moving, they quickly become cooler to the touch and clammy. All their tissues relax, and the pull of gravity results in the blood pooling to the lowest space. If you turned them at this point, you would see the back of their limbs and their back appear like a bruise, with the mottling and pooled blood at that surface. The top surface color is paler and grayer.

Rigor Mortis: This is the name for the stiffness that occurs in the body. It begins in about two hours after death. The family, staff at facilities, and hospice staff are encouraged to place the person on their back, with their arms at their sides or across their abdomen or chest, which permits an easier transfer onto the cart by the funeral staff.

Eyelids and Jaw: At death, the eyelid and jaw muscles totally relax, which means that they lay open instead of closing. If moved immediately, the eyelids may be closed and remain that way, but the jaw will not be able to close unless a scarf, which is a common item used in some cultures, is tied from below the jaw to the top of the head very tightly and done within two hours.

Calling the Agency: It is necessary to have a staff member come to do the formal pronouncement that the patient has died.

Sacred Time Right After the Death: While you wait for the staff member to arrive, settle into this amazing moment in everyone's life. Now you can relax, knowing that you did everything possible to keep them safe and comfortable. They trusted you to help them manage this transition from living with you physically to living in another dimension as a different form of energy that is no longer palpable.

At this time, many people are able to receive messages or have visions and remarkable experiences in various forms from those who have transitioned. If your family prays, say prayers. If there is another ritual common for those present, do that. If you do call the funeral home or cremation agency, they will tell you that they need to speak with the hospice staff to officially get the time of death, the name of the agency, and the name of the staff person who pronounced the death. It is very common to wait for the hospice agency staff to arrive, pronounce the death, and then call. Decide whether other family members or friends need to be called and whether that time should be right away or not.

Pronouncement at a Facility: The staff at the nursing facility will call to inform you and give you the time of death and offer condolences. They will ask whether you would like to come and be with the deceased for a while. They will offer to call the agency that has been arranged to pick up the person. Going to be with your family member is completely up to you. Some who have visited recently feel at ease about remaining at home; others will want to go, and the facility will welcome them for whatever time they need. Please note that most funeral homes request to receive the body in four hours. When the call is made to them, any specific rules of theirs will be reported.

At the Family Home: After the staff has pronounced the death, they need to make the calls to the agency, doctors, and coroner in some cases. The family or the staff can call the funeral home or cremation agency.

A staff member may have you witness the disposal of any controlled substances. The medications were ordered for the patient, and, in some states, they belong to the patient and the family. It may be a requirement for the hospice staff to dispose of them. If not, they will explain about the proper ways to dispose of medications yourselves.

If you have equipment from a hospice agency, that company will call within a few hours or the next morning to arrange to pick it up at a time convenient for the family. Other supplies are yours to keep and cannot, because of infection-control policies, be taken from the home by the staff.

When the funeral home or cremation agency staff arrives, determine whether observing their activities will be emotionally comfortable for each person in the home. The hospice staff will help them and ensure that your loved one is properly covered and gently moved onto the cart they use for transport. You can decide what you want for your last look at the amazing person who just died. You will probably witness the staff member taking a moment to honor the space and the person who just died. They might smooth the covers and say a silent prayer. This is a sacred moment for them, too.

Be prepared that during the next period of time, sometimes for just a few days until the next activity for the family happens, there may be ups and downs of belief and denial and sadness and joy and busyness and difficult-to-manage alone times. Be kind to yourself and share as much with others as you want and they want. Grieving is like dying; there are generalities to expect but no given timeline for them to occur.

Every death is unique and offers many fascinating family stories to tell. The next chapter will bring the first five chapters together in a start-to-finish lineup. For some, it will be the first chapter they read!

Chapter 6:
The Whole Picture
from Start to Finish

This chapter identifies the major points in the timeline, from deciding that hospice care is the right choice to having bereavement services available for the family. Many of the topics were addressed in other chapters, so some are lengthy while others are shorter.

Decision to Start Hospice Care

When the patient has no more curative treatment options, the doctor has a discussion with the patient and family. Sometimes, the home health nurse is already involved, or the palliative care nurse practitioner will make the recommendation. To get a good picture of the clinical status that qualifies one for hospice, the criteria that specify a major diagnosis and the qualifying additional comorbidities are listed online. Patients must be medically in a state of decline that makes a prognosis of six months or fewer pretty certain.

If the patient has been getting treatment for their condition, receiving a hospice referral is tantamount to the doctor believing that further treatment is not likely to produce a cure.

For CMS or insurance to cover hospice care, the patient must decide to stop curative treatment. Admission to hospice must be at least 24 hours after ending home health or receiving the last curative treatment. The criteria set by CMS are specific, and agencies can be penalized later during audits if they fail to comply with the regulations.

Clearly, not everyone dies within six months, but as long as one continues to decline, based on certain criteria, they continue in hospice. This happens to many patients for a few reasons. One dynamic is that the patient and family are more emotionally and spiritually relaxed, knowing there is a team watching over them. Another is because the symptoms become managed.

If the patient is already in a skilled nursing facility (SNF) or hospital, they will recommend a few agencies with which they have had good experiences. The law requires that you are given options, and you do not have to accept their recommendation. In some cases, an agency may have to get a contract written with the hospital or SNF to provide care. That's a common process despite how the social worker or medical staff may portray the situation.

If the patient is at home, recommendations may come from friends, church associates, or the person's medical staff or other medical professionals who are friends of the family.

If you have a recommendation for a specific nurse, you can call and ask for that nurse. They are assigned by geography, but exceptions are sometimes made. If that's the case, the nurse must agree to go out of their general area. Some of the staff have a large geographic area to cover, so driving 30–60 minutes between locations is entirely possible.

Sequence of Events

Order

The doctor's office or medical facility staff sends the order to the agency you choose.

Agency Acceptance

The agency evaluates the order and insurance coverage then assigns the case either to their marketing staff or directly to a nurse to start the assessment and sign-on process.

Meet and Greet

Within 24 hours of verifying the insurance, this meeting with the patient and family is done by either a nonclinical marketing staff member, in most cases, or a nurse (preferred). This is done to get consents signed, to decide the level of care (i.e., routine, continuous, general in-patient), to explain the legalities, to ask about obtaining a Do Not Resuscitate (DNR) and Living Will (so all wishes are followed), and to instruct everyone to call the agency and never 911 with a problem.

This also is a time for the staff member to ask the family and patient about a feeding tube if that has not already been done. (It may have been done in a skilled nursing facility or hospital while deciding on advanced directives.)

It is important to know that many hospice agencies will only admit people who have a DNR although it is not a CMS requirement. Signatures also are needed to get the consent for the start of care, authorize either Medicare/Medicaid or private insurance to pay for the services, assign the medical doctor (a primary care physician who will be available for consultation and eventually sign the death certificate), and explain and sign the Rights and Responsibilities forms. All those explanations are given, signatures are obtained, and the person is given a booklet that contains copies for their reference as well as very thorough explanations of many aspects of hospice legalities and care.

Funeral home information also is discussed, and if the family already has a plan, those details are given to the agency. Help will be given at both the chaplain's and social worker's first meetings, or subsequently, for finding a funeral home or crematorium, if needed. A patient's condition can change very quickly, so having this difficult discussion done right away is a priority.

The meet-and-greet staff determine whether certain durable medical equipment is needed and get that ordered, so it can be delivered prior to the patient coming home from the hospital or the skilled nursing facility. It will be delivered to a skilled nursing facility as well. The facilities appreciate the delivery of equipment because that frees up their own equipment and supplies to use with other patients.

There are three levels of care for hospice patients. Following is a brief explanation regarding who provides the care. The business and regulatory information about these levels of care is further described in Chapter 2: How the System Works.

Routine Care: If the patient is in a skilled nursing facility, that staff does all the care and notifies the hospice team about any changes. The hospice team does visits with the same frequency as if the patient were living in their own home. If the patient is at home, the family or hired caregiver does all the care in between the nurse's or aide's visits. This means that they give medications, turn the patient every 2–4 hours to prevent pressure sores, do wound care in between the nurse's visits, give respiratory treatments, change briefs, manage bowel and bladder care, change linens, feed patients who are dependent, keep the patient safe if they are mobile, and contact the agency about changes.

Continuous Care: This may be needed, but it is not very common. Usually the symptoms are managed well, and this ICU type of 24/7 nursing is not necessary. For this care, two nurses work 12 hours each in the home 24/7, or a patient is transferred to a hospital's In-Patient Unit for the usually temporary and intensive symptom management.

General In-Patient Care: This care happens in the rare instance of a patient needing continuous care right away, so they remain in that hospital. If continuous care is not needed, after a few days a transfer back home or to a skilled nursing facility will be arranged. Sometimes this critical care is needed because the patient requires medications to make them comfortable enough for the transition, and they die while on continuous care.

Admission

On this day, so many details are explained or introduced that it is overwhelming to most people. The hospice staff knows that you may not remember all that is said. Write down questions that you, other family members, or caregivers have. You may hear this many times: Some patients surprise us by dying on the day they are admitted to hospice! We believe they feel safe and will let go because the family's grieving needs will be attended to. This is true; bereavement services are offered for family members for 13 months. Feel free to call the agency, especially if the patient's condition changes soon after the nurse leaves. Be aware that some of the medications in the comfort kit (see Chapter 5) might be critically needed already! That is why they are provided on the same day. Agencies welcome your calls to ensure that both your confidence and the patient's comfort are maintained. A registered nurse (RN) is available 24/7 to speak with you.

Nurse Assessment

This is the official start of hospice care. It may include a meet-and-greet visit along with the consent signing. It is most often done within 24 hours of the referral. The start-of-care date is not official without this and the doctor's orders. It includes a full assessment of the patient's physical and psychological condition to fully decide whether the diagnosis qualifies and to make sure the patient is being admitted to the correct level of care. Then decisions are made about any medications, and explanations are given about how to use the primary care physician, the hospice medical director, and any equipment, supplies, and treatments. The nurse also orders everything that is needed from the specialty pharmacy and the durable medical equipment and/or supply agencies.

The First Five Days

In the first five days (per CMS regulations) expect visits that cover consent signing, nursing, aid as needed, and social worker and chaplain assessments. You will see the RN/case manager and certified nursing assistant (CNA) twice in that period, depending on the patient's needs and which day of the week the care starts. Weekends normally are reserved for urgent calls about a change in condition, but sometimes a weekend CNA visit will be scheduled for a new admission. Visits by the nurse practitioner and medical doctor are rare, but there are many cases in which the agency's nurse practitioner will come for a special need in lieu of the doctor. The only routine visits by these professionals are at recertification time to do a head-to-toe assessment of the patient's continued need for services.

Ongoing Care

Nurses and aides continue to make visits twice a week until a significant decline occurs and more frequent visits are needed. The social worker and chaplain make visits per a schedule that the patient and/or family has requested. That can be weekly or monthly or not at all. Hospice medical directors meet with the whole team every two weeks to review the patient's condition, all the care, and the medications as well as to consult on any questions about recertification and involvement with family.

Ongoing care can last from a few hours to several months. Understanding the symptoms of decline as well as the emotional issues patients, families, and caregivers go through is every team member's job. The social worker and spiritual counselor/chaplain also may very well be able to answer some of your medical questions. Always feel free to ask questions day or night. Never leave a question for the next day. The 24-hour hotline is not just for "hot or emergent" issues. A nurse who knows every aspect of hospice is always available. We would rather that you ask as the question arises rather than stress about it until the next day. All hospice staff feel that way about you and your loved ones as well as your need to feel safe, informed, and cared for.

Hiring Additional Help

Hiring help is often needed. As time goes on, any member of the team, along with family, may feel that it is time to hire more help. The social worker has a list of agencies to call. Some counties and religious organizations provide free services during the week for a limited number of hours or days, Monday to Friday. Other agencies are available 24/7. The family pays for this and is "the employer," so they do the interviewing and hiring. If possible, you can arrange the interviews with the nurse present, so his or her assessment skills can help you decide on the qualifications of the interviewee.

Most caregiving agencies require a minimum number of hours per day. If 24/7 care is needed, it is often less costly to split up the shifts to 12 hours per person rather than hiring someone for 24 hours a day. A 12-hour shift requires the staff member to be "on duty" the entire time. If a person stays in a home 24 hours, they need time off to eat and sleep. It then would be necessary for the family to do the care for the 8 hours that the agency staff member needs off. Many families want to be with their loved one, so hiring help for 12 hours or fewer works just fine. State-regulated agencies require the employer to provide a separate sleeping space and 8 hours off duty each day. During this time, they cannot administer medications. If you hire someone privately (not from a state-regulated organization), they may be able and willing to give all the medications and will negotiate with you about sleeping space, time off, and meals. Discuss with any member of the team whether you need just a few hours a day or 24/7 care. Again, this kind of care at home is paid for by the family or a supplemental insurance they might have.

On each visit, the nurses and aides instruct the family about all the care needs as described in Routine Care. During their visits, the nurse and aide will come and do all the care needed at that time, including changing briefs, cleansing them and applying lotions, checking vital signs, doing any wound care once a week to get measurements and determine whether a change in treatment is needed, and performing a full assessment to identify declines in any cognitive, physiological, or spiritual functions.

Knowing what to assess on each visit and being able to pick up on the often subtle clues of decline is how the nurse shows his or her expertise. Sometimes several members of a family will gather together so the nurse can explain and educate everyone at once. The family is asked to keep a notebook in the home, for both them and the hospice staff to write about a significant change, answer a question, and write a question that isn't critical and can be answered by a staff person arriving later that day. Each team member assesses the caregivers, too! Whether the patient is at a skilled nursing facility or with their family and hired caregivers in a home, we inform each other of strengths and weaknesses and follow up on questions and challenges encountered.

Some of the timeliest calls I received to tell me to stop what I was doing and get to the house right away to start the care needs for a dying patient came from the CNA, social worker, or spiritual chaplain! They know the symptoms and can describe the changes to the RN, so he or she knows what to do. They can put the caregiver on the phone so the nurse can give instructions.

All medical specialties require good teamwork, but the essence of teamwork is exemplified in the hospice specialty! Because of the intimate and timely nature of hospice care and the small number of members on each team, hospice team participation happens very often and fulfills each person's spiritual need for knowing we are critical to the success of the experience for the patient and family.

The Decline

The following describes the symptoms that occur when the patient's bodily functions shut down and what needs to be done. This period of time is called the decline.

We always must pay attention to the emotional, psychological, and spiritual needs of the patient whether they are cognitively aware or not! When they lose control and become more dependent, remember that their hearing is the last function to go. Also remember that their soul, which may be described differently in various cultures, remembers everything. Whether you believe in reincarnation or not, make sure you close the curtains for privacy, speak kindly and respectfully with every interaction, and provide the care you would expect if you were the patient. Treating everyone with dignity and respect is an essential aspect of hospice care. Sometimes we need to teach others about this.

Examples of the dramatic changes that signal decline are presented in Chapter 3. This chapter gets more specific about the most common physical symptoms that may occur. Some of these will require the nurse to visit more frequently to assess and write new treatment or medication orders. Some of these mean that certain durable medical equipment (such as a hospital bed, bedside commode, oxygen concentrator and back-up tanks, over-the-bed table, wound supplies, or oral care swabs) needs to be ordered. The intensity of the needed physical care also may dramatically change. Some of these are described in more detail in Chapter 5.

Pain

Grimaces and groans are indicators of pain and should be treated with the prescribed pain medications on a set schedule that all caregivers will follow to ensure that the patient is comfortable prior to receiving any physical care. This is covered in more detail in Chapters 4 and 5.

Decreased Appetite

A decrease in appetite may carry a highly emotional or cultural charge for people, but it is normal for all people to stop eating and drinking prior to death. The simple truth is that the body isn't getting bigger and stronger each day, so more food is not needed.

A few diagnoses include a liver function test that helps us know whether low albumin is related or not. If this is the cause (diagnosis dependent), there may be treatments available to increase one's appetite. Many times, a low albumin blood test is the marker to expect a decreased appetite, which is one of the many bodily changes signaling that life will end in a matter of weeks or months.

The gastrointestinal (GI) tract is now understood to act like a brain, sending and receiving messages to the brain in our skull. These two "brains" are in constant communication, so there may not be an obvious GI tract adjustment that triggers a change in appetite and thirst. Some believe that the soul or spirit assesses that the person is getting closer to dying. What we do know is that a biochemical signal is sent from the GI tract to the hypothalamus in the brain, which is the appetite-control center. That biochemical message results in turning down the appetite and thirst dial.

Another physiological process resulting in a decreased appetite is a dynamic involving the ability to chew and swallow. When the person has more difficulty digesting, their food-processing abilities to chew and swallow diminish, so they simply have no thirst or hunger.

This is one of the times when everyone needs to think, "Whose issue is it that our lives center around food and our family is always pushing us to eat?" At this time, pushing and prodding them to eat will only make them feel guilty for not making you happy! This decline is normal and necessitates providing other ways for a family to enjoy life. You can eat and drink in front of them, just let them engage as much as they want, knowing they should not be pressured to eat or drink themselves.

Fatigue and Sleepiness

Cancer and some neurological conditions are associated with severe fatigue. Hospice patients are simply more and more tired as their organs perform less and less of their normal functioning. Some patients with a neurological condition sleep most of the day for weeks to months prior to dying.

Breathing Difficulty

Heart and lung disease patients can require oxygen for a long time prior to even needing hospice. If they have more difficulty breathing, morphine (or its alternative) is used for symptom management along with changes in the oxygen level coming from the concentrator or tank. Another solution might be adding a nebulizer or inhaler treatment. Some very specific changes in breathing patterns are listed in Chapter 5. Some of those changes actually are not breathing difficulties but altered patterns that are expected. These are taught early and as often as necessary so everyone feels comfortable knowing what it means and whether medications can ease it.

Incontinence

Dementia patients may be incontinent for years whereas a cancer patient may never experience it. Pull-ups and tabbed briefs, and in some cases a foley catheter, are needed to maintain their hygiene and prevent skin breakdown.

Constipation

What goes in must come out or there are dire consequences! To avoid pain and distress, from the day of admission, you will hear nurses and aides ask about bowel movements. Solutions include laxative foods, pills, or suppositories. Managing bowels is as serious in hospice care as managing pain.

Weakness of Fine and Gross Motor Muscle Groups

Patients with Parkinson's, ALS, or MS have distinct changes in motor control that can last for months. If a patient suddenly falls when they were fully independent with all motor functions the day before, it's a strong signal to watch for global changes and a prognosis of possibly days to weeks for them to live. Their safety is now the primary concern and requires setting up protective equipment, including siderails, bed or chair alarms, checking on the patient more frequently, and providing a bell or monitor, so they can try to make contact when they need something.

Confusion and Disorientation

Dementia or post-stroke patients may be confused for years, but a patient with cancer or a progressive neurological disease may only get confused during the last week of their life. End-stage liver disease patients may receive a medication called lactulose to reduce the ammonia in their brain that causes confusion. The safety issues presented in the Weakness of Fine and Gross Motor Muscle Groups section all apply here.

Nausea and Vomiting

This is most often associated with some liver disorders and cancer patients. Liver disorders unfortunately carry a concern for hemorrhage. This is a unique consequence, and the nurse will explain it to the family at the onset of care. Having dark red or blue towels handy is a way to provide camouflage if bleeding occurs.

Immobility

This is usually a very late symptom in the dying process, but many patients cannot move independently at all because of trauma, disease, or stroke. Concerns here are all inclusive: pain, skin integrity, breathing, feeding, hydration, aspiration, bowel and bladder functioning, and attending to the person's psychological and spiritual needs.

Skin

The skin is the largest organ of our bodies. Some people have much more fragile skin than others, and all of us have bony prominences. Locations from head to foot to protect from pressure sores include the back of the head, tops of the ears, shoulders, elbows, wrists, thoracic spine, scapula, last few ribs, sacrum, pelvis, hips, knees, ankles, tip of toes, and heels. Pressure sores are caused by unrelieved pressure that blocks the circulation of the oxygenated blood that feeds every cell to keep it alive. Dead tissue can be as minor as a scrape and as serious as a hole in the lower back or hip that is five inches deep! All wounds are painful and, for this reason alone, must be prevented if possible.

In truth, a pressure sore is a preventable complication until the last stages of one's life when there is little to no ingestion of food and fluids. Sometimes, even with the best care and specialty beds, they may develop. Prevention requires that the skin be monitored, kept moist, and repositioned off the bony prominences so this lack of oxygen never happens. By using pillows for positioning and a turning schedule that is flexible and based on skin checks done every 2–3 hours as well as the dependence of the person to change their own position, wounds can be prevented. This topic will be reviewed by both the nurse and aide on each visit. At least three normal bed-size pillows are needed for positioning to prevent pressure sores.

Dependence on Nonverbal Signs and Symptoms

When the patient is no longer verbal, but their death is not imminent, everyone must depend on "nonverbal" symptoms (i.e., grimaces, groans, restless movements of the head and limbs, shortness of breath) and treat them accordingly. This state is expected and happens suddenly in some patients while many others gradually lose abilities, sleep more and more, and become unresponsive to the point of "actively dying."

The Dying Process

When the patient's death is imminent, which is a stage lasting anywhere from seven days to only a few hours, the nurse comes each day. The assessment includes listening to the person's heart and lungs. Sometimes they will check the blood pressure and use the pulse oximeter.

At their visits, the nurse and aide check the paper or notebook in the home used for recording their temperature, turning schedule, pain rate, administration of medications, and bowel movements. The staff will work with the family or caregiver to turn and change briefs, so the patient is clean and dry to prevent pressure sores. If necessary, a suppository is used to clear the rectum, and foley catheters may be used to drain the bladder. Pain, agitation, and gurgling medications are always given around the clock. Medications for changes in breathing and fever are given as needed.

Many patients appreciate the comfort of their favorite music. A fan can help if they are having breathing difficulties and anxiety; even unconsciously, feeling air moving over them has a calming effect. If the agency provides the complementary services of music, Healing Touch, Reiki, massage, or pet therapy, these modalities often are a huge comfort to all and actually can reverse agitation and soothe a person experiencing pain or breathing problems.

Instructions for maintaining comfort with turning and medications also continue until the patient dies. See more details and other aspects of this in Chapter 5.

Death, Transition, and Passing On

Eventually, breathing stops and the heart stops, then it is clear the person has died. This moment of realization is often met with surprise and disbelief. The family and caregivers might feel resistant to accepting it. They might recognize that although they have anticipated it for a while, knowing that it's finally happened is difficult or surprising.

Sometimes the nurse or aide is present when the patient dies, but that is not as frequent as one would imagine or the family hopes. It is a privilege to usher a person into their transition. We will say prayers with the family if that is desired before calling the funeral home or cremation agency.

If a staff member is not present, after about 5 minutes without respirations or pulse, the family makes a call to the agency. Calling 911 is not necessary because hospice staff have the authority to declare a death that is officially recognized by the coroners.

Within 1–2 hours, the staff member arrives to pronounce the death and offers condolences to the family. If desired, they call the funeral home or cremation agency for the family. Sometimes, the family has a close relationship with such a company and, of course, they can make the call themselves. However, the agency does need to speak with the staff to get the official time of death, so sometimes a second call is placed.

The staff notifies their hospice agency, who notifies each team member as well as the pharmacy and the durable medical equipment company to arrange the most convenient time for picking up the equipment.

In some instances, the family does not benefit from being in the room while the deceased is picked up by the funeral home or cremation staff. Other family members have witnessed this before and feel good about being part of those last few moments. The staff may take the opportunity to pull the sheets up and smooth the covers and pay their last respects to this sacred space once occupied by this person with whom they had a remarkable experience.

The hospice staff member who came to pronounce the death can stay with the family for as long as they need to help them process and manage their feelings. After the staff leaves, more help is available. The bereavement team will call and offer a variety of ways for the grieving family members to get the additional support they may need for up to 13 months.

In the days following the death, each team member will call to offer condolences. These calls can be cathartic for some. The calls may be the occasions for family members to ask questions they were not comfortable asking before or that came up after the person's transition. Any questions or comments about the experience are welcome. We value the feedback and encourage continued contact, knowing that there is no timetable for grieving.

The joys and sorrows about a person and their life experiences may show up for years. We all hope that we have made the hospice period comfortable for you, too, so you will continue to find value in speaking with the bereavement team.

Chapter 7:
What Makes Hospice Nursing So Special?

Hospice nursing is a fabulous job for a strong nurse committed to continuous learning and working semi-independently. It is holistic nursing because the nurses work not just with the patient and the doctor but with the full and extended family, hired caregivers, and facility staff.

Often this specialty requires the resourcefulness of finding practical solutions from products within the home, and it allows for providing complementary care modalities. It also is case management, not 8–12 hours of physical care for patients unless you work in the inpatient facilities. We supervise or manage the 24/7 care given by others.

Envision the difference between case management with traveling and being on a hospital floor, carrying a phone, and being contacted every few minutes to go down the hall to see a patient who is in need ASAP. The acute care field is the right place for many, but a slower pace called chronic care is what appeals to others. The world needs all of us.

At times, hospice nursing requires acute care knowledge and skills, but it's not all day every day. The combination suited me after I had spent my first 30 years of nursing in chronic care. The different culture and responsibilities available in hospice care are the reasons I spent so many years doing this work. We usually have our supervisor, the nurse practitioner, or our staff nurse peers available by phone when we need them, but contact with the medical doctor may or may not be as readily available—depending on the specialty of the doctor. However, they do respond within a few hours.

A big benefit to this job is the downtime between visits for you to recover from stressful situations. Going to the car in the parking lot or just finding a quiet room in the facility can provide that respite, even if you have multiple patients at one facility. Learning to manage stress is part of every job, and we can and should take the time needed to relax from the care of one patient and prepare for the care of the next one. The drive time to the next patient provides for all of that.

The hospice nurse needs to know about multiple diagnoses, the trajectory of decline, and the use of the equipment and medications as well as be comfortable with people and with teaching. Teaching the family and caregivers about the care and use of medications is the most critical aspect of this specialty. A hospice nurse must enjoy teaching concepts to both medical professionals and laypersons.

The caregivers, whether they are family members or a person hired to care for someone at the end of their life, choose to do this, too. They know that the nurse can't be there every day.

They want to make the patient's time as full of the quality of life they have lived thus far as possible. They want to provide dignity and respect and the excellent care that their loved one deserves. When they are taught well and the patient's death is peaceful, the nurse can be proud and recognize that they can feel the satisfaction of a job well done.

One of the most satisfying moments in my hospice tenure involved teaching a patient's wife to administer Lorazepam, an antianxiety medication, to her husband. She greeted me one day soon afterward with the words, "You are our Lorazepam." I knew in that moment that the medications were working, and she was calmer knowing that they had worked. She had learned well, and I received positive feedback about my ability to teach her well.

The supervisor in the hospice agency also must be a good manager and a good trainer as well. Because the nurses are not physically in the building, the supervisor frequently needs to check in with a new nurse and be able to find those excellent teaching moments, like a new admission or the report of a decline in condition that needs an extra visit or can open a topic for discussion during the team meetings.

In kind, the new nurse also must be honest and seek help often, asking for information, doing research, and building the vast knowledge base it takes to do this or any job well. There's a great deal to know. In a few years, many of these situations are experienced and provide that knowledge. For nurses with a significant amount of experience in medical surgical hospital care, it may only take 1–2 years. Others, have a great deal more to learn. A single facility may not have as many patients with a variety of diagnoses to learn about, but having a caseload mix of patients in their homes as well as facilities provides for that.

No perfect hospice agency exists, but the most important staff member to a good hospice experience is the registered nurse. In the general medical field, it's well known that the doctor is at the top of the chain of command and head of care. Although legally that's also true in hospice, the nurse is the titular head of care. In practical terms, changes often occur without a call to the doctor in that moment. As with all medical care, the nurses who are doing or supervising the 24/7 care best know the patient's day-to-day needs. Their orders include having some flexibility for dosage and frequency because nurses make decisions to change an aspect of care at critical moments all day long.

In hospice care, the doctor can be informed later in the day, in compliance with the flexibility of the original orders, that a change has been made. If the medication is already in the home or facility, that change can be instituted right away during the visit or even with a call to the family. Sometimes the nurse explains everything to the family and caregivers and then informs the supervisor and doctor later the same day. Nurses are encouraged to be independent within the scope of their license and the organization's rules. Thankfully the system has evolved, and a lot of time for providing symptom relief for the patient is saved by doing it this way.

Some nurses who enter the nursing profession later in life go straight into hospice nursing. Most longtime career nurses choose hospice care after serving in other specialties. It is important to know how you feel about being in another person's home compared to being in a hospital setting.

In the home setting, we are "guests," and the family has the final say on everything. If remaining with the in-home caregiver as long as it takes to ensure that they feel comfortable with the information feels uncomfortable for you, this is not the specialty for you. Visits can last 30–45 minutes or 3 hours, and if continuous care is needed, that time may become 12 hours. With a symptom change, there may be a new wound or a new caregiver. In these circumstances, new orders will be given and must be taught. The patient is counting on the nurse to teach the care so well that they do not have to be worried about who is doing all the care.

Choose this specialty carefully and realize how magnificent it can be to be wholly trusted by an entire family and staff in a facility for guiding them through the peaceful transition of their loved one.

Conclusion

This book was written to help everyone—patients, families, students, and professionals—navigate the complexities of the hospice programs and care.

Hopefully, this content has given you the information you need to feel more informed and empowered with the idea of hospice care. Many people in the world consider hospice care a huge privilege. We provide care for individuals and families with compassion, support, and expertise as they navigate the end of life.

For us, this is not depressing. It is an honor to be in this business that deals with the reality of death by helping others feel the same—that it is a special and sacred stage. And it is a stage we can plan for rather than fear. We do this by helping you provide as much quality as possible for the quantity of your loved one's remaining days.

References

Medicare.gov. (2023). *Hospice care*. https://www.medicare.gov/
coverage/hospice-care
This site explains hospice very well for laypersons. It is
brief and to the point.

National Hospice and Palliative Care Organization. (2023).
Homepage. https://www.nhpco.org
This is the site for an organization that helps those in the
hospice profession as well as the public learn more about
hospice.

Demystifying Hospice

Acknowledgments

In 1996, a very intuitive person told me she anticipated that I would be a hospice nurse sometime in the future. Two years later, I lived through a very bad experience with a hospice agency when my own family member died.

In the last four days with my relative, we never had a visit from any staff members, and we had no written reference materials for the use of the only medicine we had. We were not told about, or how to manage, all his end-of-life symptoms, which I knew nothing about because I had only worked on a medical surgical unit for one year 27 years earlier.

When I called the agency for help, the person asked if I had read the booklet they had provided. I was incredulous at that suggestion and was shocked that, even after my calling for help, they did not send anyone. We did not have the medications that, four years later, I would come to know how to use and absolutely never allow a patient and their family members to suffer the way my loved one and family did.

From that experience, I chose to do hospice in my elder years, ages 51–71. Prior to that, I had worked in several chronic care fields, which left me ignorant of the diagnoses and symptoms of decline and the use of several medications.

I went to the library and learned how to research and study on my own. I am eternally grateful to Loyola University's Nursing School where I got my BSN in 1971. The system's format became fresh in my mind, and I used it to learn a lot of what I needed. On-the-job training with the excellent and patient doctors and nurse managers was outstanding and filled in many blanks, but I'll admit that it took me four years to finally feel like I knew enough and did not fear new situations.

Back in 2000, they provided education every Friday. They knew they were teaching some newbies as well as experienced acute care nurses, and everyone got the anatomy, physiology, and pharmacology training necessary to work in hospice. This training was for every staff member, not just the nurses.

Chapter 7 is all about this amazing nursing specialty. I thoroughly loved what I did. I got job satisfaction every day a patient, family, or facility staff member let me know that the information I provided worked!

My first teachers were the doctors and nurse managers at Hospice of the North Shore, now known as Journey Care. The brilliant doctors who taught us so much were Dr. Martha Twaddle and Dr. Maureen McGilly. My coordinator was Celia Johnson whose patience and grace as a leader and teacher helped mellow my anxious desire to learn everything yesterday. Sam Patel, RN, the night triage nurse, walked me through what to expect and what to do with many of the on-call visits in my first few years of learning so much.

Harbor Light Hospice was a very short commitment, and the experience that stands out for me there was learning about doing continuous care.

My last 10 years were at Family Home Health Network, and my nurse managers that provided me with a very wide range of experiences were Peggy Janka, Janet Losso, Lisa Savaiano, and Carol Sotir, ANP. During our team meetings, we learned about the newest research that explained the complexity of determining criteria from Dr. Kieran Nicholson and Dr. Robert Marino. Administrative assistants Shavon Smith and Martha Escobedo were profoundly capable at managing the many nurses' schedules, coordinating new admissions, and taking crisis calls. They were the foundational rocks of kindness, compassion, and competence for the staff and the many anxious patients and families who called for help.

Thank you all for nurturing this nurse in her elder years!

I also thank Rick Vrenios who encouraged me through all the iterations of my consultant dreams and created the title for this book.

I also thank my siblings, Nick, for his copy editing of initial book chapters and offering suggestions for chapter titles; Christian, for helping me organize and focus my vision of doing hospice presentations into writing this book; and Amy, for narrowing down the varied functions of a hospice nurse to the overall concept of navigator.

I hope to continue as a teacher of hospice to people of all ages in any organization or privately with patients and/or families.

About the Author

Barbara Petersen, RN, is a student of many disciplines that inform her care. A graduate of Loyola University Nursing School (1971), she also has credentials from the Sanctuary School of Massage Therapy (2006) and is a current practitioner of Reiki (since 1996), reflexology (since 2000), and Master Hawaiian Elemental Healing (since 2004).

Professionally, from 1971–2000, she worked in various capacities in the medical fields of rehabilitation, infection control, adolescent psychiatry, utilization review, public health, and home health. While living in Colorado for a public health job, she began learning metaphysical modalities and added those to her nursing work and work with private clients.

From 2000–2020, she held a variety of roles, include six years of hospice (2000–2006), private duty nursing for handicapped teens, and hospice again (from 2010–2020).

During this time, she also went to school for massage therapy and worked as a licensed massage therapist with a chiropractor (2006–2008) and spent a year as a wellness nurse at an independent living facility.

Currently, she is a Hawaiian Healing practitioner in Arlington Heights, IL, at Sacred Ground (www.shopsacredground.com), which offers alternative health and metaphysical practices.

Since 1996, she has learned many modalities in the field of Energy Medicine. Certifications include Usui and Japanese Reiki, Reiki-ssage™, Craniosacral Therapy (both Upledger and Hawaiian), Healing Stones, Hawaiian Elemental Healing, and Remote Viewing). She has traveled to Hawaii eight times for advanced Hawaiian Healing classes.

One of eight children, Barbara grew up in Wilmette, IL. She now has two adult sons (one of whom is married) and some adorable granddogs.

Her interests also include playing the ukelele, taking Hula classes, painting for fun, and spreading the word about Hawaii Sovereignty, which is restoring the Hawaiian Kingdom.

Connect with the Author

I look forward to being a consultant to individuals or groups wanting to learn more about hospice.

- **Facebook:** @boopetersen, @hanalokahihealing
- **Email:** boopetersen@gmail.com
- **Website:** www.hanalokahihealing.com